# Lower Cholesterol

## Without Drugs

**A Practical Guide
to Using Diet
and Supplements for
Healthy
Cholesterol Levels**

*by Roger Mason*

# What they are saying about
## *Lower Cholesterol Without Drugs*

I really didn't want to change my diet, give up my bad habits or start exercising. You've shown me a way to lower my cholesterol without taking drugs or changing my life. Now, I'm taking ten different supplements not just for my high cholesterol, but for my general health.

John F., Miami, FL

I never knew there was any other way than prescription drugs. The drug I was on costs almost $100 a month, plus the doctors visits and the liver tests they kept running on me. The supplements you said to take are very inexpensive and I don't have to see the doctor all the time now. My cholesterol is much lower on these supplements than it was on the prescription I was taking.

Mary L., Parma, OH

I was overweight, ate the wrong foods, didn't take any supplements and sat around watching TV for exercise. I stopped eating red meat, butter and cheese for a start. I took some of the supplements in the book. I walk the dog every day now. I'm losing weight and my cholesterol is now normal. This is really reasonable.

Paul J., Lodi, CA

I had genetically high cholesterol and triglycerides both over 300. The prescription drugs I took didn't lower them much at all and cost me a fortune! I had pretty much given up until I read your book. I take most of the supplements and changed my diet a lot. I joined the YMCA and swim three times a week now. My cholesterol and triglycerides are now in the high normal range after only three months. I'm glad I discovered your book.

Charles A., Boston, MA

1

# LOWER CHOLESTEROL WITHOUT DRUGS

**A Practical Guide to Using Diet and Supplements for Healthy Cholesterol Levels**

YOUNG AGAIN PRODUCTS
310 N FRONT ST #150
WILMINGTON. NC 28401
(910) 371-2702 FAX ONLY
WWW YOUNGAGAIN.COM
WWW YOUNGAGAIN.ORG

by

Roger Mason

# Lower Cholesterol Without Drugs
by
Roger Mason

ISBN 1-884820-64-6
Library of Congress Control Number: 2001093348
Categories: 1. Health  2.Cholesterol
Printed in the U.S.A.

Safe Goods Publishing
561 Shunpike Road
Sheffield, MA 02157
www.safegoodspub.com
(888) NATURE-1

# Contents

# About This Book

Coronary heart disease (CHD) is the main cause of death by far worldwide. The published international research on the effects of cholesterol and triglycerides on coronary heart disease (CHD) is simply overwhelming and inarguable. *High blood fat levels are correlated with all-cause mortality* (death from every major *illness) and not just CHD! Almost forty years of research from Chemical Abstracts* (the "Chemists Bible") went into this book. The researchers of the world are basically very much in agreement that high cholesterol and triglyceride levels are the main predictors of CHD conditions. Homocysteine, C-reactive protein, and uric acid are the other three major factors.

This is a very factual book with many scientific citations and references to published studies in international medical journals. It was meant to be this way so you would know the things you read in here are truthful, honest, and accurate. No one has ever taken the last forty years of published research and condensed it down into a short, easy-to-read and understand book like this. There are many books available on heart and artery health, but most all of them simply aren't helpful at all. This is not just a book just on lowering blood fats, but one about total heart and artery health.

*A low fat diet of natural foods is the way to lower your blood fats.* Making better foods choices is the secret to a long and healthy life. Also, over thirty natural supplements are discussed in detail. Beta-sitosterol, flax oil, beta glucan, and soy isoflavones are recommended as the cornerstone of your cholesterol supplement program. In no other book are you going to read an explanation of how your basic hormones affect your blood lipid levels. Diet, proven supplements, natural hormones, and exercise are the the most important things you can do for a healthy heart and circulatory system.

Everyone who reads this book will have the ability to naturally improve their blood lipid profile, have better heart and artery health, and live longer without resorting to drugs or surgery. Prescription drugs only make you worse in the end. Nature has answers for all our health condition

# OVERVIEW

The information you find in this book can help you choose to take whatever path you like and still lower your cholesterol and triglycerides naturally without drugs, medication, or surgery. In an ideal world it would be wonderful to see everyone who reads this book to go on a natural foods diet, walk an hour a day, join a gym, avoid cigarettes, alcohol, and coffee, take about twenty supplements a day, and balance all their basic hormones. You would never need to test your cholesterol levels again.

Anyone can make continuing better choices in the food they eat every day. You can do some kind of exercise you enjoy even if it is just walking the dog a half hour a day. There are programs available to stop smoking and to stop drinking alcohol. It is easy to take at least a dozen of the proven, inexpensive, effective and safe natural supplements. You can saliva test your hormone levels and take melatonin, pregnenolone, DHEA, progesterone, thyroid hormones, GH, or testosterone where indicated. These are things anyone can do.

You can lower your cholesterol and triglycerides with no change in diet, exercise, or lifestyle simply by taking the supplements recommended herein, but that is *not* the message of this book at all. *Diet is central.* You will see very dramatic changes in your health just by making some better food choices every day, and taking the worst culprits (like butter) out of your daily fare. You can at least reduce excessive smoking, alcohol intake, or coffee consumption, if these are problems, without giving them up completely. You can find a physical activity you enjoy and take it up daily. And you can balance most of your hormones inexpensively without even seeing a doctor. You can even keep taking cholesterol lowering medication and use the information in this book to lower the dose and make it more effective. I hope everyone who reads this book will put down their medication forever. *You don't need prescription drugs in your life.*

CHD is by far the biggest cause of death in the Western world, but this doesn't need to apply to you. Please read this book and make some better choices in your life.

# Chapter 1: About Blood Diagnostics

We have fats (lipids) in our blood that are necessary for life. Vegans who eat no cholesterol whatsoever still produce it in their livers. We are only going to be concerned with total cholesterol (TC), high density cholesterol (HDL), low density cholesterol (LDL), triglycerides (TG), homocysteine (Hcy), uric acid (UA), and C-reactive protein (CRP). Total cholesterol is the most important to measure. HDL takes cholesterol from the bloodstream into the liver, while LDL takes it back into the bloodstream. Therefore we want high HDL and low LDL levels generally. Triglycerides are esters (stable forms) of fatty acids and glycerol. Obesity is strongly correlated with high TG.

You should have your blood lipids measured annually as part of your medical checkup. The usual ceiling of 200 mg/dl for total cholesterol is just too high- *150 is the realistic ideal.* (Multiply the European number by 38 to get the American number.) Most rural Asian people and vegetarians normally have levels of only about 150. This is a very practical and realistic goal. Divide your cholesterol level by your HDL level for the cholesterol:HDL ratio. For example, if your total cholesterol is 200 and your HDL is 40 (200 divided by 40) you have a ratio of 5.0. Men should be 4.0 or lower and women 4.5 or lower. Triglycerides should be under 100. You can also use the home test kits available in the drug stores, but they only give values for total cholesterol.

Every year about 1.6 million Americans suffer heart attacks and almost one third of them die. *The higher your cholesterol level the more chance you have of not only having a heart attack, but suffering from stroke, atherosclerosis (clogged arteries), high blood pressure, Alzheimer's, cancer, diabetes, and early death.*

The National Cholesterol Education Program has done a lot to tell the public about the dangers of high cholesterol. Look at the following chart *(Archives of Internal Medicine* v. 148, 1998) on cholesterol and death rates. 361,662 men aged 35-57 were studied for six years. The men with low cholesterol had only 3 deaths per 1,000 every year, while the men with high cholesterol had 16 deaths per year. *Over 500% more fatalities.* This is a huge difference, and clearly proves the diagnostic value of your total cholesterol level. All cause mortality is the gold standard.l

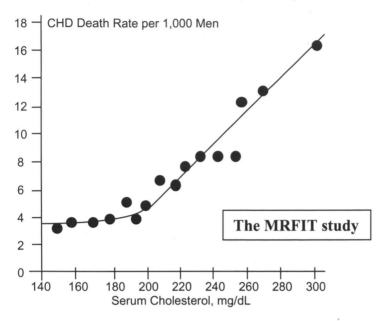

The Multiple Risk Factor Intervention Trial (MRFIT) study was based on 361,662 men aged 35-57. This was one of the largest, most important studies ever done on heart and artery health. This study has been covered in many medical journals due to the tremendous amount of information that was found. You can see for yourself here. Based on the studies of over a third of a million people the lower your cholesterol (down to a level of about 150) the longer you are going to live. *The higher your cholesterol the less time you have on earth.*

It is very important you have your amino acid homocysteine (Hcy) level tested. The normal range is 5 to 15 mmol, so you must be in the lower range here and not merely midrange. A level under 10 mmol is good. Studies show rural Mexicans, for example, with good diet had levels of 9, but urban Mexicans, with westernized diets, had levels of 12. A level over 15 is considered pathological (hyperhomocystemia). Levels over 15 cause TWICE the CHD disease rate! The higher your Hcy level the more CHD of all kinds you will suffer from. Diet and life style are the right way to lower Hcy. Whole grains lower homocysteine. You can lower this with a triple supplement of vitamin B-6 (2 mg), B-12 (as 1 mg methyl cobalamin),and folic acid (800 mcg), but this has not been shown to actually reduce CHD occurrence. In fact, at McMaster University in Canada 5,522 people were given this supplement for five years and studied. Their homocysteine went down considerably, but there was no reduction in coronary heart disease. The older you get the higher your Hcy level goes. Men have higher levels than women. Smoking, drinking coffee, high total cholesterol, and hypertension all raise Hcy. Diabetics, and those with insulin resistance, have higher levels. High Hcy is also associated with depression and dementia. Keep your level of Hcy under 10 micromoles with diet and life style.

It is very important you have your C-reactive protein (CRP) level tested. The hs-CRP (high sensitivity) test is an important inflammation marker. You want levels under 1.0 mg/liter on a 1.0 to 3.0 average range. CRP accurately predicts CHD conditions in general, as well as diabetes, and arthritis. High uric acid, hypertension, insulin resistance, smoking, high homocysteine, oral contraceptives,  high total cholesterol, obesity, lack of exercise, and high triglycerides are major factors. You lower your CRP, as usual, with diet and lifestyle. Less calories (not less food, but better food choices), more exercise, less fat (especially saturated fat), less animal protein (meat, dairy, poultry, eggs), less alcohol, weight loss, no smoking, more minerals, no birth control pills, and less sugar (any kind) intake are the ways to lower CRP. Weight loss and exercise stand out the most here. Rural Asians have very low CRP levels generally due to low fat diets and physical labor. Black Americans have higher levels generally. Again, exercise and weight loss are the two most effective ways to lower CRP.

It is very important you have your uric acid (UA) level tested. Your level should be under 5.0 mg/dl for men, and under 4.0 for women. The conventional wisdom says that foods high in purines raise uric acid. A closer analysis shows this is not the real cause. Actually, animal products per se raise uric acid levels. Red meat of all kinds, all poultry, eggs, milk and dairy products all raise your uric acid level. It's not just purines, since dairy products have almost no purines. The proof is that vegetarians, vegans, and

11

macrobiotics have far lower uric acid in their blood. Americans, who eat the most meat (due to their affluence), have the highest uric acid levels on earth. Most Asians, especially in China, Japan, Thailand, and Viet Nam, (who eat the least amount of animal products) have the lowest levels. Seafood in moderation does not raise uric acid. Sugars of all kinds also raise UA, and that includes honey and fruit juice. High UA has been clearly correlated with hypertension, diabetes, insulin resistance, metabolic syndrome, low HDL, high LDL, high triglycerides, obesity, high insulin, high blood glucose, arterial plaque (clogged arteries), arterial stiffness, and coronary heart disease in general. At the Spokane Heart Institute it was shown people with levels over 5.2 mg/dl had 3.5 times the risk of cardiovascular death! The most stunning study of all was from the Radiation Effects Foundation in Japan (*Journal of Rheumatology* v 32, 2005). 10,615 people were studied for a full 25 years. The higher their uric acid the more all-cause mortality.That simply means they died from every known cause! Men have higher levels than women. Women range from 2.4 to 6.0 mg (average 4.2) so they should be under 4.0. Men range from 3.4 to 7.0 (average 5.2) so they should be under 5.0. Do not accept average levels here.

You should know your blood sugar level and keep this under 85 mg/dl. If you suspect any blood sugar problem get an inexpensive glucose tolerance test (GTT). This shows how your cells response to insulin and is better than testing insulin itself.
High blood sugar and insulin resistance are predictive of coronary heart disease in general as well as diabetes.

Urinary albumin excretion is also well correlated with coronary heart disease. Get your creatinine checked if you get this test. Both are excellent diagnostic tools for kidney health. Kidney disease is epidemic in America and closely related to hear and artery disease.

# Chapter 2: Risks and Diseases

The published clinical evidence over the last four decades overwhelmingly shows that total cholesterol and triglycerides are the two most important diagnostic factors for overall cardio-vascular health, quality of life and longevity. Always remember CHD is the biggest killer of all by far worldwide. A review of the published medical literature for the past 40 years proves beyond any doubt that eating a diet high in saturated fats causes a rise in blood fats and resultant heart and artery disease. High fat diets, especially saturated animal fats, are a major cause of many other health problems such as diabetes, lung disease, kidney disease, pneumonia, Alzheimer's, and most all cancers. This massive evidence is based on millions of people, as well as epidemiological and migration studies. It is inarguable.

There are so many studies it is almost impossible to choose which ones to use. We'll take the reviews and the largest of the studies. One review (*Atherosclerosis* v 118, 1995) from St. Bartholemew's Hospital in London looked at ten major cohort studies around the world. They said, "A systematic examination of the evidence on the relationship between serum cholesterol and ischaemic heart disease shows conclusively that serum cholesterol reduction in populations with high rates of heart disease is an effective and safe method of reducing heart disease rates." All of these very large studies proved that the higher the cholesterol levels the more heart disease. No matter how much people lowered their levels (down to 150) there were continual beneficial effects. Again, we see that *the ideal is about 150 mg/dl.*

The MRFIT Study of 356,222 men leaves no doubt as to the facts. A chart from that study is on page 10, and shows the direct relation of cholesterol levels to heart and artery disease. This review (*Circulation* v 88, 1993) studied men from 40 different countries. This showed that CHD rates rise as cholesterol levels go over 150. This is not just a phenomenon for people with higher levels over 200. For every 1% rise in your cholesterol level you have a 2% rise in risk of coronary disease. The researchers said, "The relationship between serum cholesterol and six year risk of CHD death was continuous, graded, and strong over the entire

13

range..." This means the ideal level is about 150 mg/dl and anything over that raises your risk of CHD. They also found that beyond any doubt *diet was the major cause of high blood fats*. Dairy foods, such as milk and butterfat, were especially indicated.

The MRFIT study was also reviewed in the *Journal of the American Medical Association* (v 256, 1986). They said, "the relationship between serum cholesterol and CHD is NOT a threshold one, with increased risk confined to the two highest quintiles (groups divided into fifths), but rather is a continuously graded one that powerfully affects risk for the great majority of middle-aged American men." Again, this means that every point over a level of about 150 greatly increases your chances of heart disease and early death.

The Seven Countries Study *(European Journal of Epidemiology* (v 9, 1993) had been ongoing for 25 years in 1993. Of all the factors they said, "Over 50% of the variance in CHD death rates in 25 years were accounted for by the difference in mean serum cholesterol." Men in Japan averaged levels of about 165 total cholesterol while men in Finland, the Netherlands and the U.S. had levels of about 250! As always, the lower the level, the lower the coronary disease rate. The cholesterol level is a far more important factor than smoking, drinking, exercise, or even blood pressure.

At Providence University in Taiwan (*Journal of the American College of Nutrition* (v 118, 1999) a study was done with centarians (people 100 years of age and older) to see what factors allowed them to live so long. Total cholesterol level was one of the very most important factors for predicting longevity. Even though cholesterol levels are supposed to become less predictive as we age, this study showed that low blood lipids is always a central key to longevity regardless of how old you are.

The American Heart Association published a Special Report in the journal *Circulation* (v 81, 1990) on the importance of cholesterol as the main cause of CHD. "The evidence linking elevated serum cholesterol to CHD is overwhelming", they said. They reviewed all the major studies, especially the Framingham, Helsinki, and MRFIT since they are the largest in the world. To their credit they said that diet is the most important factor and the best solution to the problem, rather than drug treatment.

The famous Framingham Study again showed that total cholesterol, HDL, LDL, and triglycerides taken together are the single most important determinant of heart disease. We could go on quoting major studies like this, but the point is made, the proof is there, and there can be no doubts. Please look at the chart below on saturated fat consumption in 40 countries and the death rate from heart and artery disease. *Saturated fat in your diet is the main cause of high blood fat levels.*

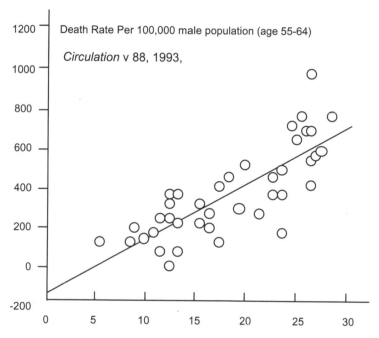

Cholesterol Saturated Fat Index per 1,000 kcal/day
The more saturated fat you eat the more coronary heart disease you get based on 40 countries.

A 25 year follow-up was done on the Seven Countries Study (Journal of the American Medical Association v 274, 1995). Here 12,467 men in seven different countries were studied for 10 years originally. "Across cultures, cholesterol is linearly related to CHD mortality, and the relative increase in CHD mortality rates with a given cholesterol increase is the same." They found cholesterol levels averaged 240 for American men, 253 for European men, but only 165 for Japanese men (this was back in 1958 and the Japanese now average about 180). The Americans and Europeans had far higher CHD rates than the Japanese.

At the National Institute of Public Health in the Netherlands (*Netherlands Journal of Medicine* v 51, 1997) doctors found that cholesterol levels increased in both men and women as they aged. In both sexes this increased an astounding 60 points from the ages of about 22 to 57. They said the main cause of this was clearly the consumption of saturated animal fats. They also agreed that many cohort studies have proven the correlation between serum cholesterol and mortality from heart disease, and this risk is continuously graded with increasing levels. After the age of 60, however, cholesterol levels tend to fall due to poor health and impaired liver function. These morbidly lowered results are misleading.

Again at St. Bartholemew's Hospital (*European Journal of Clinical Nutrition* v 48, 1994) researchers looked at international studies. The results from seventeen different countries showed, "Variations in serum cholesterol accounted for 80% of the tenfold range of CHD across countries." *In other words there was a ten times higher rate of illness and death in the higher levels compared to the lower levels.* They also said, "These results show conclusively the efficacy and safety of attaining low cholesterol levels by dietary means in lowering the risk of CHD. Policies to achieve this objective should be a major public health strategy in the economically developed world." These medical doctors said that DIET is the way to do this and not reliance on drugs.

The published international research over the last decade all come to the same conclusion. Total cholesterol, especially when used with triglyceride, homocysteine and C-reactive protein, is the best indicator we have for our risk of coronary heart disease - the largest killer by far in the developed world. Your LDL (low density cholesterol) and HDL (high density cholesterol) levels give an even bigger picture of your heart and artery health. As you might expect, people with higher cholesterol and triglyceride levels also generally have higher CRP and homocysteine levels.

# Chapter 3: Diet, Diet, Diet . . .

A wholesome low-fat natural diet is the most important thing you can do to keep your blood fats at healthy levels. *Diet is the very key to health more than any other factor.* If you were eating well you would not have a cholesterol problem. The supplements are very secondary to eating a low fat diet that is high in fiber and whole complex carbohydrates. A diet based on whole grains, green and yellow vegetables, beans of all kinds, fruits, soups, salads, and seafood will allow you to live longer and have a much higher quality of life. *Your fat calorie intake should only be 10 to 20%.* Any more than 20 percent just won't help you. The problem is that Americans and Europeans eat over 40 percent fat calories, and most of these are saturated animal fats. *It is animal foods that cause high blood lipid levels.* Asian people of most all nationalities traditionally have very low cholesterol levels, as they eat very little animal fat. In their countries the average cholesterol level is only about 150. The average American adult level is about 240. This is the main reason for our extreme CHD epidemic.

Red meat such as beef, pork, and lamb, is the main cause of high blood fats. You don't have to be a vegetarian to change this, but you do need to moderate the amount of red meat you eat. You just can't eat one-half pound slabs of red meat every day and expect to have healthy cholesterol levels. If you insist on eating meat, get the most out of it by cutting lean meat into small pieces, marinating it, and stir-frying it with lots of vegetables. You can also use small amounts in soups. Fish and seafood are much better choices, if you aren't allergic. Fish and seafood in moderation do not raise your cholesterol or triglycerides.

Poultry and eggs are two of the top ten allergenic foods known. Many people have unknown allergies to both poultry and eggs. It doesn't matter whether this is chicken, turkey, duck, pheasant, goose, or whatever. Eggs are actually worse than poultry because of the very high (i.e. 250 mg per egg) levels of cholesterol found in them. Take eggs out of your diet completely if you want to have healthy cholesterol levels. Using natural egg substitutes can be a *temporary* transition here.

Low fat dairy products are now widely available, but are still full of lactose and casein. All adults of all races are lactose intolerant and no longer secrete the enzyme lactase. Casein is a proven cancer promoter that only exists in milk products. Lactose reduced dairy products do not solve the problem, nor do organically produced ones. Organic milk is a bad joke. This is discussed in *Chapter 4: Fats and Oils.* Use soy (or almond, oat, and rice) milk, soy cream cheese, soy yogurt, and soy cheese instead of dairy. These contain vegetable oils and no lactose.To see more on this go to www.notmilk.com or www.milksucks.com. Milk and milk products are the most allergenic foods on earth.

*Whole grains should be the basis of your meals.* Whole grains are literally the staff of life, and have been for centuries. Eat brown rice instead of white, eat whole wheat pasta instead of white, eat whole grain bread instead of white, eat whole grain cold cereals instead of the refined ones, eat more oatmeal, barley, buckwheat, and cornmeal. You can eat all the whole grains you want, never be hungry, and stay slim throughout your life. Whole grains have been the staple food of most civilizations for the past five thousand years. Countless studies prove the more whole grains you eat the healthier you are and the longer you live.

Green and yellow vegetables come in a great variety. Learn to cook these fresh in variety of cultural ways by reading cookbooks from around the world. Some people think of vegetables as boring and lacking in taste because they don't know how to cook them creatively. Vegetables contain many other important and necessary nutrients besides vitamins and minerals such as sterols, lignans, antioxidants, and other vital constituents.

Beans are considered by some as "peasant food", but beans should be a basic part of our diet. Pinto, black, navy, northern, garbanzo, pink, lentils, lima, kidney, cranberry, fava, red chili, aduki, and other beans make a wonderful addition to our diets. These are full of fiber, protein, vitamins, minerals, and other nutrients. Studies show that eating beans actually lowers our blood fats. A study at Pontif University in Chile fed beans to laboratory animals and lowered their cholesterol 20% (*Journal of Nutritional Biochemisty* (v 3, 1999). Other published studies have shown beans help lower cholesterol and triglycerides.

Fruits, of course, have no fat or cholesterol, and should be eaten instead of sweetened desserts. Limit your fruit intake to about 10% of your diet. Sweeteners of all kinds eaten in excess will raise our blood fats, especially our triglycerides, due to disrupting our metabolism. A study at the University of Minnesota (*American Journal of Clinical Nutrition* v 55, 1992) showed when healthy people were given modest amounts of common sugars such as fructose, "resulted in significantly higher fasting serum total and LDL cholesterol and also caused transient change in postprandial (after meals) serum lactate and triglycerides". Honey, maple syrup, molasses, brown sugar, raw sugar, evaporated cane juice, etc. are no better than regular white sugar. *All sweeteners are basically the same simple* sugars- sugar is sugar is sugar. Raw sugar is another bad joke. Fruit juice has just as much sugar as soft drinks, and this is mostly fructose. Yes, the same fructose you find in high fructose corn syrup.

If you don't want to be a vegetarian, seafood can be eaten in moderation. Fish and shellfish do not raise our cholesterol levels, are easily digested, and are very nutritious. A few people are allergic to fish and seafood. Nuts are 90% fat calories generally, and are only to be used as a garnish. It is best to avoid Nightshade family vegetables such as potatoes, tomatoes, eggplants, and all peppers. These contain toxic solanine. It is also good to avoid the most well known allergenic foods including citrus fruits, peanuts, yeast (bakers and brewers), chocolate, and coffee.

What scientific studies do we have that eating a low-fat, complex carbohydrate diet really works? Lots of studies, and we'll go over some of them briefly. At the Institute of Biomedical Science in Taiwan (*American Journal of Clinical Nutrition* v 58, 1993) young male and female vegetarians were studied. They ate diets of 63% whole complex carbohydrates. Not only did they have consistently lower cholesterol and triglyceride levels, but their other blood parameters such as uric acid, fibrinogen, antithrombin, etc. were excellent. You don't have to be a total vegetarian to gain these advantages in your health.

Another study in the *American Journal of Clinical Nutrition* (v 83, 2006) was done at Harvard University. They stated very clearly, "Whole grain intake is inversely associated with risk of diabetes and ischemic heart disease in observational studies." The found the people who ate the most whole grains had lower cholesterol, lower triglycerides, lower blood sugar, lower homocysteine, lower C-reactive protein and lower insulin levels. They concluded, "The results suggest a lower risk of diabetes and heart disease in persons who consume diets high in whole grains."

At the University of Otago in New Zealand (*European Journal of Clinical Nutrition* v 52, 1998) young (average age 37) healthy men were given either a traditional high fat Western diet, or a low fat diet based on complex carbohydrates from grains, vegetables, legumes and fruit. The men on the healthy diet lost weight, their cholesterol levels fell, their HDL levels rose, while their LDL levels fell in only six weeks. They were allowed to select their own foods from a range of natural foods offered.

Another study in the *European Journal of Nutrition* (v 55, 2001) was done on men and women in Norway. 33,848 people 35-56 years old were studied for all cause mortality. Norwegians have a tradition of whole grain, especially bread, and eat far more than Americans. The more whole grains they ate the less disease of all kinds they suffered from and the longer they lived. They had lower cholesterol and lower blood pressure. They had fewer CHD and cancer deaths, as well as deaths from other causes.

A third study in the *European Journal of Clinical Nutrition* (v 42, 2003) showed vegetarians have dramatically lower uric acid levels. In the first chapter we discussed the importance of maintaining low uric acid levels and how eating animal foods of all kinds is the real cause of excessive levels. Some seafood, legumes and other healthy foods have considerable purines but do not raise uric acid. High uric acid is also a basic cause of kidney stones, and 10% of Americans will eventually suffer from these.

At the University of Auckland (*Diabetes Research* v 63, 2004) people were allowed to eat all the low fat food they wanted. They lowered their body weight, cholesterol, LDL, blood sugar, and blood pressure with no exercise or other changes. The more compliant they were the more benefits they got. They simply made better food choices and ate less fat.

Harvard University sponsored The Nurse's Study and did a follow up for many years. The *Journal of the American Medical Association* (September 28, 2000) reported that the 75,251 participants were questioned as to how many whole grain foods they ate. The women who ate as little as two or three slices of whole wheat bread had up to 40% less ischemic strokes (the most common form) than the women who didn't eat whole grains. *The more whole grains they consumed the more their risk of stroke declined.* This study has been going on for almost twenty years now. Strokes are the third leading cause of death in the U.S. and affect men and women equally.

The Physician's Health Study of 21,376 doctors (*Archives of Internal Medicine* v 167, 2007) found the more whole grain breakfast cereals they ate the less heart disease, hypertension, stroke, diabetes and obesity they suffered from. "Our data demonstrate that a higher intake of whole grain breakfast cereals is associated with a lower risk of heart failure."

At the USDA Human Nutrition Center (*Journal of the American College of Nutrition* v 23, 3004) men with high cholesterol were fed a whole grain based diet, including brown rice, whole wheat and barley. In merely two weeks their total cholesterol fell 20%, their LDL fell 24%, triglycerides fell 16%, and HDL rose 18%. Studies like this show just how dramatically diet lowers blood fats with no other changes in lifestyle. Adding proven supplements, exercise, and natural hormone balance would result in even more dramatic results.

Dean Ornish (*Lancet* v. 336, 1990) actually reversed clogged arteries in a year with a low fat vegetarian diet. This is thought to be medically impossible. The patients were just fed whole, natural foods with no other changes in their life styles. Dean does a lot of work in this area and has written several books on natural diet.

Not surprisingly, cholesterol and triglyceride levels are very correlated with obesity. You can easily lose weight without dieting by simply making better food choices. You can literally eat more food with less calories when you choose better foods. You do not have to eat less food at all; you just have to eat healthier foods. You do not have to count calories or adjust your portions either. The hunger drive is even more primal and more powerful than the sexual drive, and no amount of willpower will stop you from eating when you're hungry. You must fill your stomach when you eat and you can fill your stomach with delicious natural food, and enjoy your meals greatly while staying slim and feeling good.

Calorie restriction is another important factor. Americans eat twice the calories they need. You eat less calories by making better food choices. Fats contain twice the calories of protein or carbohydrates. Eat two meals a day rather than three. Don't snack. Fast one day a week on water from dinner to dinner. You will never be hungry doing these things, but can cut your calorie intake in half.

Billions of dollars are wasted every year treating the *symptoms* of obesity because we refuse to look at the *cause* of this epidemic of being overweight. Americans basically eat high fat, low bulk, low fiber, high-calorie density, highly refined, high-sugar foods. People in Asia, Africa, and Latin America generally eat lower fat, high-bulk, high-fiber, low-calorie density, unrefined unsweetened foods for the most part. If you eat a high-fat diet you will have a high body fat ratio. In fact, the very same fatty acids in your food will comprise the fat deposits in your body. Vegetable oils are just as fattening as animal fats and have the same amount of calories. You are what you eat, and the more fat you eat the fatter you will be. A stick of butter has about 1,000 calories but won't satisfy your hunger very well. In comparison, it would be impossible for most people to sit down and eat twenty apples having the same 1,000 calories. A good book to read on how to eat all the delicious natural food you want while staying healthy and slim with low blood fats is Terry Shintani's *The Hawaii Diet*. Other good books on eating well have been written by Dean Ornish, Neal Barnard, Susan Powter, Gary Null, Robert Pritikin, and any of the macrobiotic authors such as Michio Kushi.

# Chapter 4: Fats and Oils

Saturated fats are basically found only in animal foods, and cholesterol is only found in animal foods. If you didn't eat red meat, poultry, eggs, and dairy products you wouldn't have a cholesterol problem in the first place. Yes, fish and seafood contain a little saturated fat and cholesterol, but, in moderation, do not raise your cholesterol or triglyceride levels. Most people are not willing to stop eating meat, poultry, eggs, and dairy, and it is certainly their right to eat these foods in *moderation*. However, it is simply impossible for you to eat these foods as staples and maintain healthy blood lipid profiles. A breakfast of bacon, eggs, and buttered toast is simply not reasonable. You can reduce the amount of animal foods in your diet and still be happy. You can certainly take the worst of these, like bacon, butter, and cheese, out of your diet and replace them with other foods. *Ideally you want to eat 20% or less of fat calories*, and most all of these from vegetable sources. The best diet for people recovering from heart or artery disease would only be 10 percent fat calories. Reducing your fat calorie intake to, say, 30 percent is just not going to show any bene-fits. *The magic number is 20% or less.* Twenty per cent.

You may be looking at all those low-fat or no-fat dairy products out there, but they all contain lactose. Lactose and casein are the problems with dairy, in addition to the saturated fat. What is wrong with milk sugar (lactose)? After the age of about three years old all babies stop secreting the enzyme lactase, which digests the lactose. No adult of any race secretes lactase and is therefore unable to digest milk sugar. Asians and Africans especially are sensitive to dairy products. Casein is proven to promotes various cancers. *Milk is the number one allergenic food on earth.* There are a variety of very good tasting soy products you can replace dairy foods with. There are many brands of soy, rice, oat, and even almond milk. Lactose reduced milk is *not* the answer. Meltable non-dairy cheese comes in a variety of tradit-ional flavors such a cheddar, jack, parmesan, and mozzarella.

What oils are good for general use? Corn oil is a fine choice since it comes from grain. Safflower and sunflower oils are a good choice. Sesame is too expensive for general use. Olive oil is also a good choice, but olive oil is not, "good for you", no matter what you've read about it. Soy oil does not taste good unless it is so highly refined as to be nutritionless. Peanut oil comes from one of the top ten allergenic foods known and should be avoided. Cottonseed oil was never meant for human consumption and is merely sold for profit as a byproduct of the cotton industry. Walnut, avocado, almond, and other gourmet oils are expensive and have limited use in salad dressings and such. Avoid anything that is labeled "vegetable oil" or "vegetable oil blend" as these can be almost anything! Usually it is cottonseed or other cheap industrial oil in food grade. Palm and coconut oil are only for *occasional* use. These oils are really meant for the indigenous people in the hot, tropical areas where they are grown and produced.

Let's talk about canola oil. You see it endlessly promoted as a healthy oil. This contradicts the facts completely. The name comes from "Canadian oil", is from the rapeseed plant (from the Latin "rapa" or turnip), and contains less than 2% erucic acid. The normal rapeseed plant contains so much toxic erucic acid that humans and animals cannot eat the oil. The plant was extremely genetically engineered to lower its erucic acid content. Therefore it cannot be called natural in any sense of the word. Avoid canola oil and any foods that contain it, as it is purely a promotion for profit. The rapeseed plant was never meant by nature for human or animal consumption. Avoid canola.

Americans eat an astounding 42 percent fat calories, mostly saturated animal fats. Whole, natural foods supply all the essential fatty acids you need. You should take a gram (a mere 9 calories) of flax oil daily to supply omega-3 fatty acids, which are lacking in our diets. Eat as little fat in your diet as possible. It's fat that makes you fat, not food. Read the labels of every food you buy to see the percent of fat calories. Bake and broil your food and stop frying it. Stop using fats like butter to flavor your food. Read books on healthy eating by Dean Ornish, Neal Barnard, Gary Null, Robert Pritikin, Susan Powter, Michio Kushi, and Terry Shintani. You can eat all you want when you eat healthy natural whole foods like whole grains, vegetables, beans, fruits, salads and even seafood. You don't need to "go on a diet." *You just need to make better food choices.*

# Chapter 5: Trans-Fatty Acids

Hydrogenated vegetable oils actually warrant a separate chapter for many reasons. These are the worst possible fats you can eat and are even more harmful that the saturated animal fats. They are in so many of our foods, and often well hidden, that it is difficult to avoid them. As of 2006 they must be separately listed on food labels, if you get 0.5 g or more per serving. Hydrogenated oils do not exist in nature, so our bodies simply cannot recognize and digest them. People just don't realize how unhealthy these chemical abominations are, or they would quit eating countless tons of them every year. Read the labels of every food you buy and you'll be amazed at just how commonly found they are. It is very difficult to avoid them in restaurants since they are not required to list them on the menu.

Margarine is not, "better than butter", and never has been. Food manufacturers found they could extend the shelf life of foods and make them less subject to rancidity by using these cheap, artificial, man made creations. "Saturating" vegetable oils is done by subjecting inexpensive ones, like cottonseed and soy, to high pressure and heat, with hydrogen gas using exotic catalysts like platinum. This extends shelf life at the cost of your health. In this chapter we will prove to you beyond any doubt that these artificial laboratory creations are hurting your health and shortening your life. Never again knowingly buy or eat any foods containing them. There are many, many studies on the negative effects of trans fatty acids, but we will only look at a few of the most informative human ones done at some of the most prominent clinics.

At the University of Kuopio in Finland (*Metabolism Clinical & Experimental* v 48, 1999) healthy women were studied in a randomized, cross-over protocol by giving them the usual highly saturated fat European diet or diets high in hydrogenated oil. A mere 5 percent hydrogenated oil in their diet caused higher total cholesterol, LDL cholesterol, and triglyceride levels in just four weeks. They concluded the hydrogenated fat diet, "resulted in a higher total/ HDL cholesterol ratio, and elevation in triglycerides and ApoB (a negative indicator for heart health) concentrations."

At Tufts University (*Metabolism Clinical & Experimental* v 45, 1996) elderly men and women were fed either a diet of 30 percent fat calories from corn oil, or one with hydrogenated corn oil margarine for a month. They then switched to the opposite diet for a month. They said, "Mean total cholesterol levels were lowest when subjects consumed the corn oil diet as compared with the margarine diet." This is real world proof on real people that margarine raises your cholesterol levels, contributes to clogged arteries and heart disease, and causes poor quality of life, ending in early death.

At the National Public Health Institute in Finland (*American Journal of Clinical Nutrition* v 65, 1997) 80 healthy men were studied for their intake of trans-fatty acids. Half the men were given diets high in saturated animal fats, and the other half diets equally high in trans fatty acids. They concluded that high amounts of the trans-fatty acids, "had more adverse effects on lipoproteins than did equal amounts of animal fats." The intake of trans fats also worsened the LDL/HDL ratio. This is proof that hydrogenated oils are even worse than saturated animal fats.

Quite a lot of work was done at Wegeningen Agricultural University in the Netherlands. One group of researchers there (*Canadian Journal of Physiology* v 75, 1997) reviewed other major studies on the effects of trans fats on humans. They found that it is well established, "trans fatty acids raise serum LDL and lower HDL in humans." They also found that trans fats raise lipoprotein A, "Lp(a)", which is a basic indictor of heart disease. They warned that, because of their adverse effects, all foods containing them should have clear statements on the labels as to the amounts therein. This was finally done in 2006. In another study there (*Journal of Lipid Research* v 33, 1992) healthy men and women were given diets based on either vegetable oil, animal fat, or hydrogenated oils. The researchers said, "7.7% of energy from trans fatty acids in the diet significantly lowered HDL cholesterol and raised LDL cholesterol..." A third study at Wegeningen was another review of other major studies, with a full 22 references (*Current Opinion in Lipidology* v 7, 1996). The doctors came to the same conclusions as the others about the adverse effects of trans-fatty acids in our diets. Europeans and Americans are eating about 5 to 15 grams a day and the amount is rising. It should be zero grams a day.

A really impressive study was done with 748 men (*American Journal of Clinical Nutrition* v 56, 1992) at Brigham and Women's Hospital in Boston. This was a very in-depth and complex study that measured many physiological parameters and biological markers. It was clear to the doctors that trans-fats in our diets raise LDL levels, lower HDL levels, and raise total cholesterol. They said, "On the basis of results from other studies...this would correspond to a 27% increase in the risk of myocardial infarction (heart attack)." Trans-fats in your diet equal heart disease and outright heart attacks.

Some fine research was done at the University of Oslo in Norway (*Journal of Lipid Research* v 36, 1995) where young men were fed either margarine or butter in their diets. We've been told for many years now that, "margarine is better than butter", when, in fact, it is worse than butter. The men eating the margarine lowered their HDL levels, which made their HDL/LDL ratio worse. The researchers concluded, "consumption of partially hydrogenated fish oil may unfavorably affect lipid risk factors for coronary heart disease..." You don't need to use butter or margarine.

*At the famous Harvard Medical School (Lancet* v 341, 1993) doctors reviewed the very large and long term Nurses Study of 85,095 women and how much margarine and hydrogenated oil they reported consuming. It was obvious that the intake of these fats was, "directly related to risk of coronary heart disease", and that "consumption of partially hydrogenated vegetable oils may contribute to the occurrence of CHD." That's pretty clear.

Some very alarming work was done collaboratively at several clinics around the world working together to study breast cancer *(Cancer Epidemiology Biomarkers Preview* v 6, 1997) They studied 698 cases of breast cancer in European women and concluded that, "the adipose concentration of trans-fatty acids showed a positive correlation with breast cancer." This means they actually took biopsies (tissue samples) of breast tissue to analyze how much hydrogenated fats were actually in the bodies of the women from their dietary consumption. Now we have a proven link in humans showing the relation of eating unnatural trans-fats to higher cancer rates.

At Limburg University in the Netherlands (*Journal of Lipid Research* v 33, 1992) doctors studied the effects of trans-fats on levels of lipoprotein A, aka Lp(a), which they called a strong risk factor for CHD. There were three strictly controlled experiments on healthy men and women fed either saturated fats, monosaturated and polyunsaturated fats, or hydrogenated oils. Those people on the hydrogenated oil diet raised their Lp(a) levels to very dangerous levels in only a month. They concluded, "These short-term experiments suggest that diets high in trans-monosaturated fatty acids may increase serum levels of Lp(a)." If this was done in a month imagine what the effects are year after year.

From time to time you will see studies in medical journals, such as a recent 2001 issue of the *Journal of the American* Medical Association, claiming that these hydrogenated oils are very safe, or even preferable to natural fats and oils. Back to the old, "margarine is better than butter" story. You will notice in small print in each of these so-called "studies" that they are funded and paid for by organizations such as the United Soybean Board and the National Association of Margarine Manufacturers. So much for objective science. Unfortunately, you can purchase space for your advertising-posing-as-science in many medical journals.

Folks, read your labels. Stop buying any foods that contain hydrogenated or partially-hydrogenated oils. Do not eat in fast food restaurants as nearly everything they serve is full of these. You can find such things as potato chips and corn chips that aren't made with hydrogenated oils. You can temporarily use non-hydrogenated margarines such as Smart Balance®/Earth Balance® from your grocery store. You will be surprised at just how many foods contain these unnatural and dangerous synthetic oils. In 2006 the FDA finally required all food products to state prominently the trans fat content of their product on the front of the label. If a food has hydrogenated or partially-hydrogenated oils in it don't buy it and don't eat it. When you eat out ask the manager what kind of oil they use in the kitchen. Actually trans-fats shouldn't even be allowed in our foods at all.

# Chapter 6: Practical Supplements

This will be the longest chapter in order to cover all the clinically proven effective supplements. These will be in alphabetical order. Always remember supplements are secondary to diet in lowering cholesterol and triglycerides and improving CHD health.

**Acetyl-l-carnitine** (ALC) is a much more effective form of l-carnitine. Take 500 to 1,000 mg a day. This is also very important for brain metabolism and maintaining good memory and clarity of thought as you age.

**Acidophilus** is important to keep our intestinal flora (good bacteria that digest our food) in balance and prevent growth of the harmful bacteria. It is in our large intestine where fats are digested. This is where cholesterol is either absorbed or excreted. Various studies have shown that acidophilus is also good for cardiovascular health. Purchase a good refrigerated brand with at least 6 billion units per capsule containing several different strains, and keep it refrigerated. You can use a special, stable spore form called "lactospore" along with regular acidophilus for even better results. People in Western societies usually have very low counts of good bacteria due to eating too much food, too much fat, too much protein, drinking coffee and alcohol, and eating too much sugar. These cause poor digestion and the many resulting problems. Be sure to take FOS and L-glutamine with your acidophilus for best effect.

**Alfalfa** extract has been promoted for lowering cholesterol, but there doesn't seem to be any published studies on this in the last twenty years. Alfalfa is a fine herb, but is relatively weak and needs to be extracted. This does not seem to be a good choice.

**Alginate** (sodium alginate) is an effective, natural seaweed extract. It is very effective for lowering blood lipids and removing toxic heavy metals like mercury, lead, and cadmium from our blood. Scientists have known about both of these qualities for decades now, but it never became a popular supplement for some reason. It is not easy to find this at the retail level, so just

29

Google "sodium alginate". This is an inexpensive, safe, and very overlooked way to lower your cholesterol. Take about 3 grams a day for one year, as it is exogenous.

**Artichoke** leaf extract contains chlorogenic acid, cynarin, and other effective compounds. There are a few studies that showed if you took enough of it you could lower your cholesterol. Artichoke extract is well known for its beneficial effects on the liver and in treating liver ailments. This is pricey and almost no one offers it, so it is not a practical choice currently.

**Beta carotene** is a good antioxidant to take, and will work with other supplements synergistically to lower cholesterol. Take 10,000 IU daily of any good brand. This is a better choice than taking vitamin A, and has many other benefits for your health generally. There are many studies on beta carotene showing how powerful and effective it is as an antioxidant, how it helps regulate cholesterol metabolism, and protects against atherosclerosis. This should be a part of your daily supplement program for many other reasons than just lowering cholesterol.

**Beta Glucan** is discussed in Chapter 10.

**Beta Sitosterol** is discussed in Chapter 8.

**Carnosine** (L-carnosine) is an amino acid that helps support good heart health. It reduces glycation (sugars binding to proteins) and has antiaging properties. It is found in our muscles basically. Animal testing has shown great potential here, and human testing has verified some of this. Take 500 to 1,000 mg a day. There is lots of good science here. Since CHD is the biggest killer by far, this is important for anyone over 40.

**Chitin** is the natural fiber found in shellfish shells, and has been sold as a popular diet aid since it absorbs fat, especially saturated fat, in the food we eat. This will help lower cholesterol if you take about 2 grams a day. Use only for one year. Most of the diet products sold actually contain chitosan (an unnatural, synthetic derivative) instead of real, natural chitin. Always choose the natural product over the synthetic one when you can.

**CoQ10** is a very heart healthy supplement. Take 100 mg and no less. *Buy real Japanese uniquinone and not ubiquinol.* Take your CoQ10 with food or flax oil for best absorption. All "special delivery systems" are scams. Levels fall as we age, and this is not found in food. This is a very important supplement for anyone over the age of 40. This is very important for total cardio-vascular health.

**Curcumin** is the active ingredient in the spice tumeric. This has been used in Indian Ayurvedic medicine for over 1,000 years. Curcumin is a very impressive supplement with antiviral, anti-inflammatory, anticancer, and antioxidant effects, as well as in cholesterol lowering ability. Take at least 500 mg of actual curcumin as stated on the label. There are lots of good studies on using curcumin for lowering cholesterol. This is exogenous, so only take it for six to twelve months.

**Vitamin C** is a fine antioxidant *when used in moderation of 250 mg or less a day.* We only need about 60 mg. Taking megadoses acidifies our naturally alkaline blood and unbalances our system. Long term studies show the dangers of using megadoses. *Limit this to 250 mg.* Claims are always being made that taking several grams a days (3,000 to 5,000 mg) will result in great health benefits. All of these are wrong! Studies prove that taking such doses result in much more debilitating side effects than benefits.

**Vitamin D** cannot be emphasized enough. This is not found in your food and most people do not get out in the sun enough to synthesize it. *Deficiency of vitamin D is epidemic especially as we age.* Be sure to take the 400 IU in your vitamin supplement as well as an extra 400 IU (unless you are out in the sun regularly). Avoid overdoses as this is fat soluble.

**DIM** (di-indolylmethane) is important to help keep estradiol and estrone levels low. High estrogens in men or women are harmful to heart health. Take 200 mg. All "special delivery systems" are scams.

**Vitamin E** is a definite for heart and artery health. Forty years ago the medical world would not even admit vitamin E was

31

a necessary nutrient! This is found in whole grains and is very deficient in our diets. Take 200 IU of any good brand you like, but be sure to choose the natural, mixed tocopherols, not synthetic d-alpha. People with heart problems can take 400 IU. 400 IU will tend to thin your blood. The studies on vitamin E and CHD health go back 40 years and are overwhelming. This is definitely one of the basic supplements you want to take daily. Your multivitamin will most probably only contain the RDA of 30 IU.

**Fenugreek** extract has shown some promise in lowering cholesterol due to its galactomannon fiber content, but the few animal studies used very large amounts to do so. Until there is good human research this is not a good choice.

**Fibers** generally, especially psyllium, are very good for keeping your cholesterol low and they will also help keep your bowel movements regular. You can use sea fiber like chitin, or the usual plant fibers like guar gum, glucomannon, fruit (apple or citrus) pectin, oat bran, wheat bran, or others. Ideally your diet should be full of fibers especially from whole grains and various beans. *Eating a naturally high fiber diet is the best way to get your daily fiber intake*, rather than taking a supplemental form.

**Flax Oil** is discussed in Chapter 9.

**FOS** is short for fructooligosaccharides, otherwise known as inulin, an extract of chicory root. This has been known about for a long time, but only recently was it discovered that this feeds your good intestinal bacteria. The higher your levels of beneficial flora in your intestines the lower your cholesterol levels generally. FOS is very good for your intestinal health, and has good science behind it. Anyone with intestinal disorders should consider using this in large doses (like 1.5 grams twice a day) for a year. FOS is widely available and you should take one or two 750 mg capsules a day with your acidophilus. Take FOS along with a refrigerated brand of acidophilus and some L-glutamine every day. Abstinence from alcohol and coffee, a low fat/low sugar/high fiber diet, and eating lower calorie whole foods will improve your digestion greatly.

**Garlic** has many proven health benefits. Human studies over the years have verified the advantage to garlic supplements for better cholesterol levels. Here it is important to get a good, reliable brand with high levels of active ingredients stated on the label. If you take an unknown brand you may well get few results. Of course, you can choose to use fresh garlic in your daily cooking. The composition of garlic supplements varies greatly so you have to get a good reliable brand to obtain results.

**Glucomannon** is a plant fiber from the konjac root and may help you eat less while lowering your cholesterol. It is inexpensive and widely available. You should take at least 2-3 grams a day prior to meals. It swells up in your stomach giving you a feeling of fullness so you may eat less and still feel full. There are many studies, including human ones, on the effectiveness of glucomannon. Take this for just one year.

**Glucosamine** is very important for bone health. This needs co-factors such as calcium, magnesium, boron, silicon, and vitamin D. 95% of Americans over 65 are arthritic.

**Glutamine** is a common amino acid known as L-glutamine. It is easily found and very inexpensive. L-glutamine has shown very impressive benefits for intestinal health. Progressive surgeons are giving it to their patients after intestinal surgery. It also has been shown to spike levels of human growth hormone when taken in doses of one gram two times a day (AM and PM). The scientific literature has recently published many studies on the benefits of L-glutamine supplementation. This is a definite part of your supplement program and will help keep your intestines full of good bacteria and free of the bad bacteria.

**Glutathione** is one of the two basic antioxidant enzymes that help fight dangerous free radicals and are involved in cholesterol metabolism. Ironically, taking oral glutathione does a poor job of raising blood levels. Fortunately there is a supplement called N-acetyl-cysteine or "NAC" that effectively raises glutathione levels. Take a 600 mg NAC capsule daily. Unfortunately, the other basic antioxidant enzyme, S.O.D. (superoxide dismutase), is not absorbed orally, and must be injected to get into the bloodstream. Doctors do not have injectable S.O.D. yet. NAC is a good general supplement for anyone over the age of 40.

**Grape extract** can come either from the seeds or from the skins. Grape *skin* extract is known as resveratrol and is useless. The "studies" are paid ads. Do not waste your money on resveratrol. The *seed* extract is a popular and effective antioxidant, but there is just no real proof it will help lower cholesterol levels.

**Guar gum** is a very good fiber to use. It is easier to take in capsules as mixing this with any liquid will thicken it up so much it will be hard to drink. In fact it is commonly used in very small amounts as a thickener in foods such as salad dressing. There are many studies on the benefits of this fine fiber from the Cyamopsis plant in India. Like other such fibers you need at least 2-3 grams a day for results. Surprisingly, there are lots of studies on this natural supplement. It is inexpensive and widely sold. Take for one year as this is a good choice.

**Guggul Gum** is a fine exogenous supplement you can take for 6-12 months. Take 250 mg of 10% extract so that you get 25 mg of actual guggul sterones. Not only does this help lower cholesterol and triglycerides, raise HDL, and lower LDL, but also lowers uric acid. Human studies have shown up to a 15% drop in total cholesterol, and a whopping 26% in triglycerides with no change in diet or exercise. Not everyone will get such dramatic results however. Admittedly there is a lack of published science.

**Lecithin** emulsifies dietary fats so they can be digested more easily. It works by decreasing the absorption of cholesterol in our intestines, and by other mechanisms. This soybean extract is sold everywhere and is very inexpensive. Take a 1,200 mg softgel daily. It is also known as phosphatidyl choline and is good for brain health, memory, and liver function. (Do not confuse it with "PS" or phosphatidyl serine, which is also a fine supplement for brain health in 100 mg doses.) This is a good choice for good heart and artery health with studies going back for many years. Lecithin has been shown to lower total cholesterol, LDL cholesterol, and homocysteine levels, as well as being anti-atherogenic and helping keep our arteries clear of fat buildup.

**Lipoic acid** blood levels fall as we age. This is not found in your food. Take 400 mg of regular R,S-lipoic acid to maintain low blood sugar levels. R-only lipoic acid is a scam. High blood sugar is strongly associated with coronary heart ailments as is insulin resistance. Keep your blood sugar under 85 mg/dl.

**Magnesium** is a vital mineral that deserves separate mention since it has many proven benefits. Magnesium should definitely be a part of your supplement program, as calcium cannot be absorbed, without magnesium, boron, strontium and silicon. Even if you are eating a diet rich in whole grains (the best source) it is still wise to take about 250 mg daily. There are numerous scientific studies on magnesium supplements that show various benefits to health including lower cholesterol and even lower blood pressure. Make sure your mineral supplement contains this. Magnesium does not work alone and must have all the other basic nineteen minerals with it.

**Minerals** are very important to every aspect of our health. The importance of getting all the minerals and trace elements we need for proper cholesterol synthesis and metabolism is not generally recognized. We are all mineral deficient in some way. Mineral deficiency is linked to every health condition known. You need about 20 elements including calcium, magnesium, iron, zinc, boron, selenium, chromium, iodine, molybdenum, manganese, copper, germanium, strontium, nickel, tin, cobalt, rubidium, cesium, silicon, and vanadium. More research needs to be done in this area. Google "mineral supplements" to find only one (the one your author developed of course) with 20 elements. Read the label to make sure the *amount* of each mineral is clearly stated. Minerals are covered in detail in Chapter 8: The Minerals You Need. You can also read my book, *The Minerals You Need*.

**Niacin**, niacinamide and "non-flushing" niacin overdoses are NOT good choices for lowering your cholesterol, regardless of the hype you've read. You don't need massive doses that unbalance your metabolism, even though it is a water-soluble vitamin. You only need 20 mg a day. Remember that *megadoses of anything unbalance your body and hurt your health.*

35

**Phosphatidy serine** (PS) is an important supplement to take for brain health. This works well with ALC and pregnenolone. Take 100 mg a day. A well proven supplement for cognition, memory, clarity of thought, and to prevent senility.

**Policosanol** (aka octacosanol) is an outright fraud. All the "studies" come from a storefront in Cuba posing as a clinic. In 2009 claims are even being made for heart health and other benefits. Anytime you see some self-appointed authority on natural health promote this you know they are clueless. Don't waste your money. Who else on earth is warning warning you about scams like policosanol, lycopene, and resveratrol?

**Pectin** is found basically in the inner rind of citrus fruits and in apples. All are very effective. Do NOT fall for the advertisements for overpriced "modified" citrus pectin. Modified pectin is an expensive fraud. Plain old, regular, inexpensive citrus or apple pectin is a very effective fiber. Like the other fibers, you need to take at least 2-3 grams daily. Studies abound on the use of pectin, and this is a very good choice when you take enough of it. There are other health benefits to taking pectin. Take for one year. It is a good, safe, proven, and effective supplement.

**Red rice yeast** has been promoted as a wonder drug for cholesterol. There is almost no science here, and it hasn't been proven to be safe. Supposedly this contains a "natural version" of a statin drug. This is reason enough not to use it!

**SOD** (superoxide dismutase) is the second antioxidant enzyme. Our levels fall as we age, and low SOD levels have been consistently correlated with high blood lipids. The problem is that there are no practical SOD supplements. It must be injected, and doctors do not have SOD or even know about it. It is not legal to prescribe it sublingually or as a nasal spray. The oral SOD tablets sold are a scam. Real SOD is biosynthesized and costs $1,000 a pint. You can find topical SOD creams, but these are not transdermal and won't raise your blood levels.

**Soy Isoflavones** are discussed in Chapter 11.

**Spirulina** has been hyped for a long time now as some kind of wonder food. It is simply fresh water algae as is chorella. There are no valid studies in the last 30 years on any benefits from taking spirulina, much less to lower blood fats, and no active ingredients were ever identified.

**Taurine** is a common amino acid that can be used temporarily to help lower our blood fats. There are also benefits for diabetes and other blood sugar conditions. Take 500 mg for one year even though it is endogenous and found in our daily food and in our bodies.

**Tea (green)** really does work and will help your cholesterol levels. The catechins and polyphenols found in green tea are very powerful antioxidants. Find a decaffeinated brand and do not take the inexpensive brands that are full of caffeine. This is simply common black tea before it is fermented. Many studies have been done on the health benefits generally and the active ingredients. Green tea extract is a good choice for a lot of reasons. Take this for only one year, as it is exogenous and not a common food.

**TMG,** aka trimethylglycine, aka betaine, has powerful rejuvenation properties for our liver. The human studies on this are most impressive. Take 3 grams of this every day for six to twelve months to cleanse and strengthen your liver. After a year take 1 gram a day for maintenance and lower Hcy levels. Our livers are stressed from our high fat diets, our intake of prescription drugs, recreational drugs, alcohol, coffee, and preservatives. The liver is our largest internal organ and processes the fats in our blood. *The liver and gall bladder are central to cholesterol metabolism.* This is very important to do! Take TMG to rejuvenate and cleanse your liver.

**Vitamins** only number thirteen, and there is an RDA for each of them. You can easily find a complete vitamin formula with all thirteen in the recommended RDAs. Find one with 1 mg of methyl cobalamin instead of regular B-12 as it is much more absorbable. Regular oral B-12 simply does not get into your bloodstream.

If you are over 40, or have a medical condition of some kind, there are temporary, exogenous (not in your body or your food) supplements you can also take for your general health. **Quercitin** (100 mg) is a strong antioxidant well worth taking. **Aloe vera** gel (200:1 extract) is a fine temporary supplement that can be used for up to a year since it is exogenous. Take two 100 mg capsules. **Milk thistle** extract (2 capsules) is another temporary supplement that can be used for up to one year to cleanse and tone your liver. **Ellagic acid** (100 mg) is a temporary supplement that has shown anti-cancer and other properties.

We now have children with high cholesterol and triglycerides for the first time in human history. Children and people under 40 don't need many supplements. They can take beta glucan, flax oil, acidophilus, FOS, L-glutamine, a good mineral supplement, a good vitamin supplement, vitamin D, and vitamin E. An 80 pound child would need half doses, and a 40 pound child quarter doses. This would apply as well for your pets; a 20 pound dog would only need eighth doses.

Do not waste your money on such promotional frauds as lycopene, chondroitin, nattokinase, noni juice, colloidal minerals, sea silver, colloidal silver, coral calcium, hoodia cactus, resveratrol, 5-HTP, deer antler, modified citrus pectin, saw palmetto, Pygeum africanum, maca root, chrysin, MGN-3, AHCC, oral S.O.D., megadoses of *anything*, whey protein, Gymnema sylvestre, MSM, 7-keto DHEA, evening primrose oil, horny goat weed, tongkat ali, tribulis terrestis, coconut oil, bilberry, pomegranate products, arginine, cat's claw, brewers yeast, shark cartilage, ginger root (for arthritis), oral hyaluronic acid, cranberry juice capsules, DMAE, CLA, goji berries, OTC (over-the-counter) growth hormone secretagogues, OTC testosterone boosters, acai fruit, mangosteen products, *any weight loss product*, *any* sexual rejuvenation formula, all bee products, all homeopathic products, and other such useless promotions. Please read my book *The Supplements You Need* for more information.

# Chapter 7: The Minerals You Need

Science has shown how important minerals are for any disease or medical condition. *Every single health problem known is due in part to mineral deficiency.* We're all mineral deficient no matter how well we eat. There are only ten elements officially classified as essential with an RDA set for them. There are at least twenty four elements we need. We get sufficient sulfur, potassium, phosphorous, and sodium in our daily diet. The best mineral supplements sold in the world only contain about ten elements. There is only one supplement that has all twenty (from yours truly). Just google "mineral supplement" on the Internet and you'll find it. Read the label, and look at the amounts contained in the product. Colloidal minerals, coral calcium and the like are all useless scams.

**Calcium** is the most abundant element in our bodies, and 99% is found in our bones. It is essential, of course, but the RDA of 1,000 mg is simply not scientifically sound at all. Only dairy products contain large amounts of calcium, and you shouldn't be eating them. 400 mg would be a much more reasonable figure. There is little problem with calcium intake; the real issue is absorption. Calcium needs co-factors such as magnesium, boron, strontium, silicon, and vitamin D in order to be absorbed and make bone. There is too much emphasis and research on calcium and not enough on many of the other minerals.

**Magnesium** is the fourth most abundant element in our bodies, with an RDA of 400 mg. Americans only eat about 300 mg, so deficiency is common. A supplement of 200 mg a day would be fine. Common salts are good. The main source is whole grains, but we only eat about 1% whole grains now. Magnesium is the center of the chlorophyll molecule, which is the life blood of the plant world. There is massive research on magnesium, and this is a very heart healthy mineral.

**Iron** is one of the ten essential elements, and deficiency is as common as ever. Even with our excessive consumption of red meat and animal products (the most abundant source) many people just don't absorb what they need. . Copper is needed for absorption and there is an important iron to copper ratio. Iron is occasionally found in high levels in hyper-cholesterol conditions, but this is due to an excretion problem and not excessive intake. Iron retention and lack of excretion fortunately is a rather rare problem. Iron is the "heme" in hemoglobin, and the basic mineral in our blood. Iron is the center of our red blood cells, and this is why it is so important. You shouldn't be eating red meat, so you won't have to worry about overconsumption. A good supplement will contain the female RDA of 18 mg. The male RDA is only 10 mg. Common sulfates, fumarates, and gluconates are good.

**Zinc** is one of the ten essential elements. Most of the zinc in the male body is found in the prostate gland. This may be either high or low in those with high blood fats; there is just no consistency here. Most people do not get the 15 mg RDA they need from the food they eat. There is an important zinc to copper balance. Zinc is found in whole grains, beans, nuts, and meats. Deficiency is especially true for the poor, elderly, and alcoholics. There are about 2.5 g of zinc in the human body, almost half of which is in the muscles. Whole grains and beans are the best source. Never take in more than 50 mg of zinc daily, as the toxicity level is low. The usual citrates, oxides, and sulfates all work well.

**Boron** is definitely *the most deficient mineral in our diet.* There is no official RDA, but 3 mg is the suggested daily intake .It wasn't until 1990 that boron was even accepted as essential! The research is overwhelming here. Our soils and food are very boron deficient. You would think all vitamin and mineral supplements would contain 3 mg of this inexpensive and vital element, but very few do. This proves the mega-corporations have huge advertising budgets, but no research departments. Americans probably only take in a mere 1 mg a day. Be sure you get this in your supplement, as boron deficiency is all too common. Citrates or common boric acid is fine here. There is good science behind boron.

**Manganese** is essential, and the RDA was only recently established at 2 mg. There are a mere 20 mg in the average human body. Whole grains are a major source, along with beans and legumes, nuts, and root vegetables. Most people do get enough, especially vegetarians. There is an abundance of re-search about the benefits for our health. A supplement is still good insurance for such an important element. This is found in most mineral supplements. Threre are too many uses to list, but arthritis and bone problems are one important area of study. Sulfates and oxides are effective.

**Copper** is essential, and also has an RDA of only 2 mg. There is only about 150 mg in  the human body. As a heavy metal this can be toxic at only 15 mg a day, but that is very unlikely. Americans probably only take in about half this amount.  Studies have shown low copper is common with high blood fats.  Whole grains and beans are the best source. The refined foods we eat cause common deficiencies. There is an important zinc-to-copper ratio. Taking a 2 mg  supplement is good insurance. The known biological uses of copper are far too numerous to list. Citrates, oxides, and gluconates are all very absorbable.

**Silicon** is the ignored or "orphan mineral," and almost never found in mineral supplements. More proof that mega-corporations have no research departments, only advertising budgets. There is no RDA set for this, but 10 mg a day is a safe and effective dose. Do not use horsetail as a source. Silica levels in our foods vary so greatly, that it is all but impossible to say which foods are good sources. Bone and joint health depend on silica as a basic building block. The science here is most impressive.  Plain silica gel (silicic acid) is a good, effective, inexpensive source. You aren't going to find this in supplements except the one mentioned at the beginning of this chapter. This is one of the two non-metallic elements we need.

**Iodine** is very important, and the only other non-metallic element we need to supplement. It is essential ,and the RDA is a mere 150 mcg (micrograms). Eating sea vegetables regularly like kelp, nori, and hijiki, as many Asians do, is not a good idea surprisingly. All seaweeds  contain extreme amounts of iodine. Overdoses of any mineral unbalance your metabolism, and are not merely excreted without effect. The most important value here is thyroid metabolism. There are only about 30 mg in our bodies, and three fourths of it is in our thyroid gland. Only 30 mg.  Iodine supplements will not correct low T3 or T4 levels, or  any thyroid problems however.

**Chromium** is essential, and only recently has an RDA of 120 mcg. This is often deficient in our diet to refining the grains we eat.

This is critical for normal blood fat levels, as well as proper blood sugar metabolism. One reason for the epidemic of diabetes and insulin resistance is the widespread deficiency of chromium. Some studies estimate that 90% of Americans are, in fact, deficient. This is usually found in mineral supplements. Never exceed an intake of more than 400 mcg. Do not listen to advertisements claiming their form of chromium is the "only effective one". Regular chelates (a non-metal ion bound to a metal ion for better absorbability) are the best source.

**Vanadium** was ignored until very recently, and there is no RDA for it, even though it is not accepted as essential. Taking 1 mg (1,000 mcg) a day is good, but almost no supplements contain this vital mineral. Do not exceed one or two mg a day, as this is toxic in excess. Vanadium has been shown to be important for cholesterol metabolism. Deficiency is all too common, due to our intake of refined foods. There is now very good science on the importance of vanadium, especially for blood blood fats and blood sugar dysmetabolism. Chelates and sulfates are your best choices here. Make sure you get at least 1 mg a day.

**Molybdenum** is essential, and has an RDA of 75 mcg, but that may not be enough. Be sure to take a supplement here to insure adequate intake. All common salts are good sources, and you will find this in all your supplement formulas. Molybdenum is safe and non-toxic, even though it is a heavy metal. The research is concerned more with soil and plants, rather than animals and humans. Farmers and gardeners commonly use this in their fertilizer and animal feed.

**Selenium** finally has been classified as essential, and has an official RDA of 70 mcg. It was almost ignored until very recently. This is very deficient in our soils and heavily refined foods. Do not exceed a daily intake of more than 200 mcg, as this is a heavy metal and will accumulate in your body. Whole grains are the very best source. Chelates are the most absorbable form of selenium. Be sure to take this with 200 IU of natural, mixed vitamin E, as they are very synergistic and work together well. Studies show people with low blood selenium suffer from higher disease rates such as cancer, coronary heart disease, and diabetes.

**Germanium** is a very important ultra-trace element and you will just never find this in mineral supplements. Look for the only one in the world that has it. You only need about 100 mcg of ultra-trace elements like germanium. Do not exceed this amount, as 100 mcg is sufficient. Clinical human blood studies prove this is a vital element we need, but our soils and our food are deficient, and it is not found in supplements. Germanium sesquoxide and chelates are safe, but germanium dioxide is not.

**Strontium** is another very important trace element, with very good science behind it. You will not find this in mineral supplements, and 1 mg (1,000 mcg) is a good dose. Bone and joint health depend on strontium as a building block, as does calcium absorption. No RDA has been set, but science finally recognizes this as essential. Do not confuse this with the radioactive form strontium-90. Chelates and asparates are good choices. Look for the one supplement that has 1,000 mcg.

**Nickel** is an ignored ultra-trace element, and 100 mcg is all you need. Food and blood analysis of animals and humans show this is an essential element, but there is little research on the benefits, or for the problems caused by deficiency. The research is mostly for soil and crops. Nickel is essential in human and animal nutrition. You won't see this in the mineral supplements on the market either. Regular salts such as chlorides and sulfates are good.

**Tin** is also ignored as a necessary ultra-trace element. 100 mcg is a good dose. Common food and soil studies prove this is an essential element. Most of the research has been concerned with tin toxicity from industrial pollution, instead of the benefits. The FDA irrationally limits the dose to 30 mcg. You almost never find this in mineral supplements. Human studies have shown low blood tin levels in some illnesses, but more research is needed. Regular salts such as chlorides and sulfates are well absorbed.

**Cobalt** in never found in mineral supplements, even though it is the basic building block for vitamin B-12. Food and blood studies prove its importance. We are supposed to synthesize our own B-12, but cannot without cobalt in our blood. We probably only take in about 25 mcg or less, but that is enough. This may not sound like much, but we only need to make about 3 mcg of B-12 daily.

Taking B-12 orally just doesn't work, so you should take 1 mg of methyl cobalamin. It must be emphasized that sufficient B-12 is just not found In foods, it is orally unavailable, and a cobalt supplement should insure the synthesis of the 3 mcg you need every day. There is good science behind cobalt even in this tiny amount.

**Cesium** is an important ultra-trace mineral, and 100 mcg is all you need. Do not take more than this. Human blood, common food, and soil studies prove how vital this is for our health. You will never find this in mineral supplements. International studies show the importance of cesium in our soil, our food, and our blood. Cesium is essential for humans and animals. Soon science will admit this and set an RDA. Regular salts, especially chloride, work well here.

**Rubidium** is not an ultra-trace element at all, as our intake is about 1 mg (1,000 mcg). Taking a supplement of 500 mcg of this is enough, since common rubidium deficiency has not been demonstrated. Never found in mineral supplements (except one), and very ignored by science. Found abundantly in soil, crops, as well in mammals and humans. The few studies we have are very positive. Brain levels of rubidium fall as we age. This is definitely required in human, animal, and plant nutrition. Rubidium is found in fruits, vegetables, poultry, and seafood. Rubidium chloride is a good form to use.

Just remember that we need ALL the known minerals and not just the most well known of them. All minerals work together harmoniously as a team together in concert.

# Chapter 8: Beta-sitosterol

*If there was only one supplement you should take to normalize your cholesterol it should be beta-sitosterol.* 300 to 600 mg doses of mixed sterols every day will do wonders for you. If you have a more serious problem you can take three capsules a day, or 900 mg, but only for a year. Beta-sitosterol is the safest, most studied, proven, and effective single way known to lower total and LDL cholesterols. The studies on this in the medical journals actually go back 50 years, yet most people have never even heard of it. The published human research is just overwhelming here, and every year more studies are done on plant sterols.

What is beta-sitosterol? It's a phytosterol, or plant alcohol, that is literally in every vegetable in our diet. We already eat this every day, but just don't get enough of it. The typical American is estimated to eat only 200-400 mg a day, while vegetarians probably eat twice as much. This is surely one of the many reasons vegetarians are healthier and live longer. Actually, the term "beta-sitosterol" in commerce refers to the natural combination of beta-sitosterol, stigmasterol, campesterol, and brassicasterol, as this is how it is made by nature in plants. There are no magic foods with high levels of phytosterols, but these can be inex-pensively extracted from sugar cane pulp or soybeans.

Upjohn Pharmaceuticals tried to make a semi-synthetic, patentable, prescription analog (chemical relative) of it decades ago, but did not succeed. The natural molecule works best. The scientific community has been well aware of plant sterols, and has done extensive studies on both humans and animals. This includes gall bladder, bile, and liver functions, since these are all part of the cholesterol metabolism. The major theory of its effectiveness is in simply preventing dietary cholesterol from being absorbed in the intestines, where fat is digested. Another way it seems to work is by increasing the flow of bile acids. This binds cholesterol in the digestive tract, and excretes it in the feces. There are just too many studies to count, so a few of the most interesting human studies have been included here.

45

At McGill University in Montreal (*Canadian Journal of Physiology* v. 75, 1997) doctors did a review of the literature on beta-sitosterol and cholesterol metabolism, and selected 18 studies. They concluded that, "the addition to diet of phytosterols represents an effective means of improving circulating lipid profiles to reduce risk of coronary heart disease." This review came complete with forty high quality references and left no doubt about the effectiveness of plant sterols. Also at McGill University (*Metabolism Clinical & Experimental* v. 47, 1998) patients on a fixed diet were given sterols from pine oil for a mere ten days in a strict, randomized crossover study. These were not low-fat or low-cholesterol diets at all. The patients successfully lowered both their total cholesterol and LDL levels in this short term placebo controlled experiment. The doctors concluded, "These results demonstrate the short-term efficacy of pine oil plant sterols as cholesterol lowering agents."

A very interesting study was done at the Center for Human Nutrition in France (*Annals of Nutrition & Metabolism* v. 39, 1995) in that healthy people with *normal* cholesterol levels were given beta- sitosterol to see if their *normal* levels could be lowered even further. We always, of course, think of studies as using unhealthy people with pathological cholesterol levels, given supplements to bring them to normal again. Amazingly enough, the healthy people lowered their normal cholesterol levels even more, with no change in diet or exercise. In fact, their levels were a full 10 percent lower in only a month. This kind of effect is really fascinating. They said, "The present results may be of great interest in the prevention of high cholesterol diet-associated risks, especially in the prevention of cardiovascular diseases". Since beta-sitosterol was so effective for people who didn't even need it, think what it will do for those people who really do need to lower their blood lipids. They concluded, "These findings suggest that a significant lowering of plasma total and LDL cholesterols can be effected by a modest dietary intake of soybean phytosterols."

A good study was done at the Wageningen Agricultural Institute in the Netherlands, the same clinic that did so much good research on trans fatty acids (*American Journal of Clinical Nutrition* v. 72, 2000). Men and women ate a margarine containing plant sterols and got very significant reductions in cholesterol, as well as lower LDL levels, in only three weeks. Why a clinic would give margarine to people after studying the negative effects of hydrogenated oils is another matter. Again, these were healthy subjects with normal cholesterol levels, yet they still got great benefits very quickly, with no change in diet or exercise.

At Uppsala University in Sweden (*European Heart Journal,* Supp. 1, 1999) the doctors wanted to give the volunteers the phytosterols in conjunction with a cholesterol lowering diet to see the results of a more comprehensive lifestyle program. The results were really impressive in that the men and women lowered total cholesterol a full 15 percent and LDL cholesterol a full 19 percent, in less than a month. This shows the very dramatic results you can get by just adding some reasonable dietary changes even without any exercise program at all. All in just 30 days.

So called "complimentary medicine" doctors have learned adding phytosterols to their usual prescription statin drugs makes the drugs far more effective, and the toxic dosages can be lowered. This is NOT the point of this book at all. Complimentary medicine is an oxymoron. You can't go right and left at the same time. Statin drugs are so dangerous that liver function tests must be given periodically to make sure the liver isn't damaged too much. People with liver problems cannot take these drugs.

At the University of Kagawa in Tokyo, two studies were done. The first was done on healthy young men who were given plant sterols for only five days. In this short time their cholesterol levels fell measurably (*Joshi Eiyo Daigaku Kiyo* 14, 1983). The second study was done on healthy young women (same journal v. 15, 1984) again giving them plant sterols for only five days. "Administration of phytosterol (mainly sitosterol) increased the fecal output of cholesterol." These were all healthy young Japanese people eating a traditional low-fat diet who did not have a cholesterol problem to begin with, yet they received significant and measurable results in only five days.

At the University of California in San Diego men were isolated in a hospital ward and fed 500 mg capsules of pure cholesterol along with beta-sitosterol supplements (*American Journal of Clinical Nutrition* v 35, 1982). This resulted in a 42 percent decrease in cholesterol absorption in the intestines. They said, "Evidently, the judicious addition of beta-sitosterol to meals containing cholesterol-rich foods will result in a decrease in cholesterol absorption with a consequent decrease in plasma cholesterol." A very well done study.

The University of Helsinki took a big interest in lowering cholesterol with plant sterol therapy, back in 1988. The first study (*Clinical Chimica Acta* v. 178) studied familial (genetic) hypercholesteremia. The higher the sterol levels they found in the patients blood the more cholesterol was excreted, rather than absorbed. The second study was in 1989 (*Metabolism Clinical & Experimental* v 38). Men were again studied for blood levels of sterols and they found the same phenomenon. The third study in 1994 (*American Journal of Clinical Nutrition* v 59) studied vegetarians, who eat about twice as many plant sterols as normal people. They showed that one reason vegetarians have lower cholesterol levels is the efficiency of their cholesterol excretion due to their intakes of plant sterols. Genetically high cholesterol was again dramatically lowered in families by simply feeding them mixed sterols (*Journal of Laboratory & Clinical Medicine* v 143, 2004). The last study in 1999 (*Current Opinion Lipidology* v 10) said, "Plant sterols may be useful for the treatment of hypercholesteremia...they may have a potent cholesterol lowering effect as shown in normal and hypercholesteremic men and women with and without coronary heart disease and diabetes mellitus."

The famous Brandeis University, doctors gave sterols to men in a crossover study and lowered total cholesterol 10% and LDL a full 15% in only four weeks, with no change at all in diet. (*Journal of Nutrition* v 134, 2004). Imagine the results if they had also adopted a low fat diet. This is amazing and proves you don't need toxic drugs to lower blood fats.

The best published review of all was from the University of British Columbia (*American Journal of Medicine* v 107, 1999). This included a full 86 references, and went over sixteen different human studies that used plant sterols to lower cholesterol and triglycerides since 1951. "In sixteen recently published human studies that used phytosterols to decrease plasma cholesterol levels in a total of 590 subjects, phytosterol therapy was accompanied by an average 10% decrease in total cholesterol and 13% decrease in LDL cholesterol." They found this worked best with high-fat diets; the worse the diet the better the results the researchers got. This is the best review to date. In 2004 the same university (*Nutraceutical Science* v 1) did a sixty-three page review "Role of Plant Sterols in Cholesterol Lowering".

At the University of Calgary the researchers found (*Canadian Journal of Cardiology* v. 17, 2001), "...it is clear that phytosterols, when added to a prudent diet, will lower serum total and LDL cholesterol. Numerous well designed studies have documented the beneficial actions of these phytosterols on serum cholesterol." They point out that either sterols or stanols (relatives of sterols) are each effective. Their estimate is that most Westerners eat less than 300 mg of plant sterols a day, which is in agreement with other researchers.

Both healthy and hypercholesterolemic Japanese men were given sterols in mayonnaise for 12 weeks (*Journal of Oleo Science* v 53, 2004). Both groups significantly lowered their total cholesterol and LDL, with no change in diet or exercise. More proof that cholesterol lowering drugs are completely unnecessary.

At Washington University in St. Louis (*American Journal of Clinical Nutrition* v 77, 2003) plant sterols from wheat germ were given to patients in muffins. "The present study shows that phytosterols intrinsic to wheat germ are biologically active and have a prominent role in reducing cholesterol absorption."

At Iowa State University (*American Journal of Clinical Nutrition* v 76, 2002) men were actually given beef in their diet along with plant sterols for four weeks. This was not the ideal food obviously. "Phytosterol-supplemented ground beef effectively lowers total cholestserol and LDL cholesterol and has the potential to become a functional food to help reduce the risk of cardiovascular disease."

At the University of Rome (*British Journal of Nutrition* v 86, 2001) people were given a special low-fat, low-lactose yogurt drink with soy sterols for four weeks. "The yogurt enriched with plant sterols significantly reduced, in a dose-dependent manner, serum total cholesterol and LDL cholesterol levels. A low-fat yogurt based drink moderately enriched with plant sterols may lower total choleseterol and LDL cholesterol effectively."

At TNO Nutrition in the Netherlands (*European Journal of Clinical Nutrition* v 57, 2003) volunteers were given a vegetable spread with 1.6 grams of plant sterols for one year. This increased the sterol concentration in the red blood cells and serum (the plasma will not dissolve sterols). "Consumption of a plant sterol esters-enriched spread in an effective way to consistently lower blood cholesterol concentrations and is safe to use over a period of time."

At the University of California Davis (*Arteriosclerosis and Metabolic Research* v 24, 2004) healthy subjects were given sterols in orange juice for eight weeks with great success. "Sterol orange juice supplementation significantly decreased total (7.2%), LDL (12.4%) and non-HDL (7.8%) cholesterol compared with baseline and with placebo orange juice. Remember these were healthy people with no elevated blood fats.

We could go on all day with published studies like this from well known clinics and hospitals around the world. The research is so extensive and wide ranging over the last 30 years, that it is hard to find and count all the studies. How something so studied, proven, effective, and well known to the scientific and medical communities has stayed outside of public knowledge is hard to believe. You will notice that the expensive, prescription, patented, cholesterol drugs are the primary means to lower cholesterol. There is just no profit in a natural, unpatentable, non-prescription plant extract. If you check vitamin catalogs it still is not easy to find good beta-sitosterol supplements with realistic amounts of sterols. You can find inexpensive brands containing the 300 mg you need if you look around, or search the Internet under "beta-sitosterol".

Many studies have been done in other areas of illness that found beta-sitosterol has great potential in many conditions such as prostate disease (read my book *The Natural Prostate Cure*), diabetes, blood clotting, ulcers, cancer prevention, tumors, immunity, inflammation, and other conditions. You will see more research and more benefits for beta-sitosterol every year.

# Chapter 9: Flax Oil and Omega-3 Fatty Acids

It is very basic and important to understand that *we eat far too many omega-6 fatty acids, and too few omega-3 fatty acids.* We should have about a 4-to-1 ratio, but actually have about 20-to -1. This imbalance increases inflammation. There have been countless studies published on the benefits of omega-3 supplementation. This includes diseases and conditions of all types and not just blood lipids. It is very difficult to get a good supply of omega-3 fats in your diet unless you eat a lot of fatty fish like sardines, salmon, herring and mackerel. This is obviously not the answer. Most of the studies have, in fact, been based on fish liver oils. However, the best source in the world is flax seed. *Any studies using fish liver oils would have gotten the same results with flax oil.* Fish oil has dangerous arachidonic acid, and is more subject to oxidation. Flax is a cleaner, much tastier, less expensive plant product that is preferable to fish oils. It is the best source if vital lignans of all foods. *Buy it, and store it, refrigerated* or it will oxidize. You can also use freshly ground flax seed in your food. The omega-6 fatty acids are known as linoleic (LA), while the omega-3s are known as linolenic (ALA). Flax is the best source of ALA, which converts in the body to both DHA and EPA. Flax is also the best source of lignans in the world. Let's look at just a few of the human studies using omega-3s to not only lower cholesterol and triglyceride levels, but to improve other important blood parameters generally. More studies using flax oil rather than fish oil will be appearing in the future.

At the University of Toronto (*American Journal of Clinical Nutrition* v.69, 1999) flaxseed lowered undesirable LDL cholesterol levels in both men and women. At the National Institute of Nutrition in India (*Nutrition Research* v 12, 1992) people were given high content omega-3 oils in their diets, and their TC and TG levels dropped while other blood qualities were improved as a side benefit. At PSG College in India (Indian Journal of Nutrition v 42, 2005) elderly people were given flax oil. This lowered their total cholesterol, LDL, and triglycerides. At Nikea Hospital in Greece (*Atherosclerosis* v 167, 2003) people lowered their CRP levels with flax oil. They also lowered inflammatory markers such as IL-6 and amyloid A.

51

At the University of Iceland two different groups of Iceland-ers were studied- native and Canadian. Even though the native Icelanders had higher total cholesterol and high LDL levels (but lower triglycerides) they had far less mortality from ischemic heart disease because they had lower omega-6 fatty acid levels, yet three times the omega-3 levels than the Canadians. This low ratio of omega-6 to omega-3 fats in their blood protected them from heart disease and premature death.

At Aalborg Hospital in Denmark (*Lipids* v 29, 1994) volun-teers were given flax oil (high in omega-3s) or corn oil (high in omega-6s) in their diets in a classic double blind study. The people given the flax oil based diet lowered their triglycerides and LDL levels as well as their total cholesterol levels with no change in what they ate or how much they exercised. At the University of Oslo in Norway doctors gave fish oil (high in omega-3s) or corn oil (high in omega-6s) to different groups of people for four months. Those people getting the omega-3s lowered their LDL levels significantly and improved their other blood parameters generally.

At Ulleval Hospital in Norway (*Scandanavian Journal of Clinical Laboratory Investigation* v 54, 1994) another classic double blind study was done with 57 patients. All had high chol-esterol levels, and had undergone heart bypass surgery. Those patients given the omega-3s lowered their triglyceride levels sig-nificantly, but also improved their glucose homeostasis (i.e. their blood sugar metabolism was normalized).

At the University of Regensburg in Germany 35 men with heart disease were given a double-blind study for vegetable based omega-3 fatty acids and fish oil based omega-3s. Both groups lowered their total cholesterol and LDL levels. This is an excellent study that demonstrates whichever the source, fish or flax, the benefits still occur equally. Flax is the better source though.

At the Northern General Hospital in Britain (*Lipids* v 27, 1992) 365 people with diagnosed heart disease, high cholesterol, or a family history of heart disease were given a fish oil sup-plement high in omega-3 fats. There were no other dietary changes for a period of four full years. The ones getting the omega-3 supplement suffered a mere 1 percent of heart attack rate during this time, while the ones who got no supplement suffered a drastic 9 percent heart attack rate. *This is a 900% difference!* This proves the long term effects and how the benefits accrue over time. The fish oil group lowered their total cholesterol, lowered their triglycerides, raised their HDL levels, and lowered their undesirable blood fibrinogen levels as well. Flax oil would have been better.

At the Jordan Heart Fund Foundation in New Jersey (*American Journal of Clinical Nutrition* v 12, 1993) doctors gave flaxseed and vitamin E supplements to patients with hyper-cholesterolemia for three months. Both their cholesterol and LDL levels fell. Platelet aggregation decreased to more desirable levels, and other blood measurements were improved.

Postmenopausal women at the University of Oklahoma were given ground flax seed for three months in a double blind study (*Journal of Clinical Endocrinology* v 87, 2002). They lowered both their total and LDL cholesterol by 6.0 percent with no change in diet or exercise. They lowered their triglycerides a whopping 12.8 percent with no other treatments. This is most impressive.

It is very difficult to reduce blood pressure in people simply by using natural supplements. Generally, the only way to lower blood pressure is to make basic changes in lifestyle including diet, overall hormone balance, exercise, and reducing alcohol, coffee, and smoking. Studies show that about one fourth of Americans have high blood pressure. Now, more younger people suffer from this every year. At the University of Trondheim in Norway, doctors gave omega-3 fatty acid supplements to men with high blood pressure with no other treatments or changes in their lifestyles (*Proceedings of the Scandinavian Symposium on Lipids 16th*, 1991). Amazingly enough they lowered their blood pressure just from taking the omega-3 supplements. This kind of study is most significant. Hypertension causes strokes and early death and is very correlated with insulin resistance. Hypertension is an epidemic in the Western world.

At Nycomed Pharma AS in Norway (*Journal of Optimal Nutrition* v 2 1993) 52 men were given either fish oil (with 66 percentt omega-3 fatty acids) or olive oil supplements, for three weeks. Fibrinogen levels fell 13 percent, triglycerides fell an amazing 28 percent, and their HDL levels went up 10 percent. *The men on the olive oil increased their triglycerides a full 27%.* So much for the, "olive oil is good for you" story. The lower all the fats in your diet, the better. Vegetable oils are just less harmful.

At the University of Kansas (*Journal of Applied Nutrition* v 43, 1991) healthy men were given fish oil omega-3 supplements. Their triglyceride levels dropped an impressive 36 percent. What prescription drug at any price could give results like that? At Kings College in London (*British Journal of Nutrition* v 68, 1992) healthy males were given fish oil capsules for six weeks. LDL levels fell. Other blood parameters, such as platelet aggregation and Ap-B, were also improved. In addition, both their systolic and diastolic blood pressure levels fell. Again we find omega-3s have the power to lower blood pressure with no change in lifestyle.

At Uppsala University in Sweden volunteers were given fish oil supplements, or a placebo, for two weeks in a double blind study. Then the groups were switched and the ones getting the fish oil then got the placebo (*Nutrition Research* v 12, 1992). Regular measurements of their blood were continually taken. Dangerous Lipoprotein-A (Lp-A) was lowered by 19 percent, total cholesterol fell, as did triglycerides, and HDL levels rose in the supplemented groups. You could hardly ask for anything better than this from an inexpensive, natural food supplement.

At the Women's University in Japan 50 healthy young women with no heart or circulatory problems were studied for a wide variety of diets ranging from 15 to 40 percent fat calories. Their diets literally and directly determined the quality of their blood, especially the ratio of omega-3 fatty acids to omega-6 fatty acids they ate each day. The women with the highest levels of omega-3s and the lowest levels of omega-6s had the lowest TC and TG levels and the highest HDL levels (*Nippon Eiyo* v. 49, 1996). This shows direct blood measurement compared to diet, in normal people, and why we should eat less fat and oils

Flax oil really is amazing. This is a supplement for everyone including you children and pets. *You must buy and keep it refrigeratred.* Take 1-2 capsules or ½ teaspoon of liquid (1.5 g).

# Chapter 10: Beta Glucan

Beta glucan is the most powerful immune system stimulant known to science, including any pharmaceutical drugs, like interferon-alpha. Please read my book *What Is Beta Glucan?* It is a polysaccharide found in oats, barley, yeast, and mushrooms. The miraculous powers of beta glucan to lower cholesterol and triglycerides and strengthen our immune systems have been known about for more than a decade now. At the University of Hamburg in Germany it was shown that *all 1,3 configuration beta glucans have the same biological potency whether they are derived from oats or yeast*, which are the two major sources (*Carbohydrate Research* v 297, 1997). *They are all basically true 1,3 beta glucans.* Do not listen to advertisements that tell you one is better than the other in order to sell their product. You need at least 200 mg a day of actual glucan to be effective. You can now get 60 capsules for only $10. You can take twice this much for a year if you are treating a health condition. It has only been since the year 2000 that technology finally provided inexpensive, strong beta glucan to consumers.

Beta glucan is the most powerful immunity enhancer known to science regardless of cost. There are many studies on animals and humans, that show the great value it has to strengthen our immune systems, and even the potential to help against tumors and cancer growth. At the University of Saskatchewan in Canada (*Microbiology & Immunity* v 41, 1997) researchers showed its power to stimulate the immune system. Other studies have found such potential uses as fighting infections, improving intestinal flora, irritable bowel syndrome, diabetic conditions, healing ulcers, and better digestion. There are many, many studies on blood lipids, so we'll just talk about some of the more interesting human studies.

At Harvard Medical School in Massachusetts (*Critical Reviews in Food Science & Nutrition* v 39, 1999) doctors found that both oat and yeast beta glucans lowered serum cholesterol levels with no change in diet. In their words, "In addition to decreasing the intake of total fat, saturated fat, and dietary cholesterol, blood serum cholesterol can be further decreased by dietary fiber, especially from sources rich in beta glucan such as oats and yeast."

At the University of Syracuse in New York 71 men and women with high cholesterol were given various combinations of low fat diets or regular diets, with and without oat beta glucan. In four weeks, total cholesterol levels were reduced as much as 17 percent and HDL levels increased (*Journal of the American Dietary Association* v 90, 1990). This shows the benefit of making better food choices, along with taking proven supplements.

At the University of Massachusetts (*American Journal of Clinical Nutrition* v 70, 1999) researchers found that giving yeast beta glucan to obese men with high cholesterol lowered both their total and LDL levels by a full 8%, with no change in diet. They summarized the study, "Thus, the yeast derived beta glucan fiber lowered the total cholesterol concentrations and was well tolerated." As usual, the "side effects" were all positive in nature.

At the U. S. Human Nutrition Research Center in Maryland (*Journal of Nutritional Biochemistry* v 8, 1997) people were given oat beta glucan and lowered their cholesterol levels, with no changes in diet or exercise. They also found that other metabolic conditions improved, so new benefits of beta glucan are always being discovered. Again at the Human Nutrition Research Center (*Journal of the American College of Nutrition* v 16, 1997) men and women with high blood lipid levels were given oat beta glucan in a crossover study. After only five weeks the groups were switched, and those getting the beta glucan just received only the usual American diet. Both total cholesterol and LDL levels decreased significantly. In their words, "A significant dose response due to beta glucan concentration in the oat extract was observed in the total cholesterol levels." A third study was done there (*American Journal of Clinical Nutrition* v 80, 2004) with barley beta glucan. This lowered the subjects LDL and total cholesterol. Thorough studies like these with real people at the most prestigious research centers in the world leave no doubt about the power of beta glucan to lower blood fats.

At Industrial Research Limited in New Zealand (*Carbo-*

*hydrate Polymers* v 29, 1996) researchers used barley derived beta glucan to try and understand the actual metabolic mechanisms by which it lowered blood fats. They discovered that it increased the secretion of bile acids from the gall bladder. At the Netherlands Maastricht University (*American Journal of Clinical Nutrition* v 78, 2003) people were given oat beta glucan and lowered their cholesterol in only three weeks. Another study there, in the same journal (v 83, 2006) got identical results. Again at Maastricht (*Journal of Nutrition* v 137, 2007) oat beta glucan lowered total cholesterol and LDL levels in four weeks. Hyper-cholesterolemic children at Radiant Research were given beta glucan to get dramatic improvements in only four weeks (*Nutrition Research* v 23, 2003). At the University of Minnesota (*Nutrition Journal* v 6, 2007) men and women were given oat beta glucan for 3 weeks. Total and LDL cholesterol were significantly reduced. *JAMA* published two studies (v 265, 1991 and v 267, 1992) where adults were given oat beta glucan and lowered their cholesterol in weeks with no change in diet or exercise.

At the University of Lund in Sweden (*Annals of Nutrition & Metabolism* v 43, 1999) 66 mildly hypercholesterolemic men were given oat milk high in beta glucan every day for five weeks. This was a classic double blind study where half the men received rice milk with no beta glucan. Of course the men getting the oat milk lowered their total cholesterol, and the doctors said, "It is concluded that oat milk has cholesterol reducing properties." They did another study (*European Journal of Clinical Nutrition* v 59, 2005) and gave oat glucan to patients. This improved their cholesterol as well as their glucose metabolism, in just eight weeks.

You can see from studies like these, there is no doubt that beta glucan is a safe, effective, powerful, proven, and inexpensive way to lower your cholesterol levels, yet most people have never even heard of it. Many vitamin companies don't even sell it. It can be difficult to find a reliable, strong, inexpensive brand with 200 mg or more, even in the health food stores. Just Google "beta glucan" on the Internet to find a good brand. Many people insist on taking dangerous, expensive, prescription drugs when they can use natural remedies like beta glucan. The use of statin drugs now is epidemic.

In addition to the benefits we've just covered, beta glucan strengthens our immune system, so we have optimum healing power in our body to fight off infections of all kinds. You should understand that it is very difficult to study human beings for immune function. Animal studies are used because you just can't infect humans with deadly micro-organisms, give half of them beta glucan, and see who lives and who doesn't. Animal studies have shown results for such conditions as various cancers, infections, tumors, diabetes, digestion, intestinal function and ulcers. Finally, since 2000, we are seeing many human studies published where real people can safely be used.

At the University of Saskatchewan, beta glucan protected mice from deadly injections of Staphalococcus aureus. In another study there mice were injected with equally deadly Eimeria vermiformis, but beta glucan protected them. In a third study, mice were given the toxic drug dexamethasone and then injected with the deadly Eimeria virus. Even after their immune systems were impaired by the drug the beta glucan protected them. At SRI International the Euglena gracilis virus was injected into various test animals, but beta glucan stopped them from dying. At the University of Kansas pigs were given deadly Staphalococcus suis but beta glucan saved them. The doctors there did an in-depth study of various immune system markers to discover the mechanisms by which it worked.

At the Mayo Clinic lung cancer in mice was reduced by beta glucan. At Tokyo College, doctors found strong anti-tumor properties for beta glucan. At Tokyo University, doctors found anticancer activity in mice, when given beta glucan, and suggested it be used as a biological response modifier in human cancer patients. At Wuhan University, doctors found powerful anti-tumor activity in mice given beta glucan. At the University of Louisville, they found the anti-tumor effect of beta glucan was largely due to enhancing beneficial natural killer (NK) cells. Please read my book *"What Is Beta Glucan?"* for more information. This is a proven basic supplement for children and adults. Even your pets should be taking this daily for the same reasons

# Chapter 11: Soy Isoflavones

Surprisingly, this chapter is not going to try to persuade you to eat more soy foods. Eating more soy foods is a fine thing to do, but it is not a practical way to get sufficient isoflavones into your diet. It just isn't realistic to tell Americans to eat a lot of tofu (a highly refined food anyway), tempeh, annato, seitan, soy sauce, soy flour, soy sprouts, boiled soybeans, soy cheese, and soy milk. You could drink an eight ounce glass of soymilk every day, but that would add 120 unneeded calories every day. (This would come to 44,000 unneeded calories a year.) It's better to use it for your cold cereal and in cooking, than as a beverage.

The two main isoflavones we are concerned about here are genestein and daidzein. These are not "phytoestrogens" as you have been told endlessly. There is no such thing as plant hormones. They are, in fact, *flavones* and completely unrelated to estrogen or any other hormone. Flavones are plant pigment flavonoids, while estrogens are steroids secreted by the endocrine (ductless) glands in animals. There are countless studies on the benefits of isoflavones for most every medical condition, and new ones appear in the journals every week. We are going to look at some of the most impressive human studies that show value in improving blood lipid profiles. There are many other reasons to take isoflavones, and they should be a basic part of your supplement program. You need about 40 mg a day, so read the label on your supplement carefully. See that you are getting a total of at least that much combined genestein and daidzein.

At the Panum Institute in Copenhagen (*American Journal of Clinical Nutrition* v 69, 1999) people were given soy protein which lowered their LDL levels while raising their HDL levels in only six weeks with no change in diet or exercise.

At Baylor College in Houston (*American Journal of Clinical Nutrition* v 68 Supp, 1998) subjects were given soy protein which, again, lowered their LDL levels while raising their HDL levels in only five weeks. It was interesting to note that in this study both normal people and patients with high cholesterol levels were included, and both benefited significantly. It is difficult to get people with normal levels to reduce them even further. Even better results were obtained when the soy supplement was used with the National Cholesterol Education Program Diet, which emphasizes low fat, high fiber, and complex carbohydrates.

At St. Michael's Hospital in Toronto (*Metabolism & Clinical Experiments* v 48, 1999) men and women were given a low fat diet with added soy protein. Researchers found the soy supplement very much strengthened the effects of the low fat diet. In their words, "A combination of vegetable protein and soluble fiber significantly improved the lipid-lowering effect of a low saturated fat diet."

At the University of Illinois (*American Journal of Clinical Nutrition* v 68 Supp, 1998) postmenopausal women were given soy isoflavones. They lowered their TC levels while raising their HDL levels and lowering their LDL levels. This was a very well done and professional study. In addition to improving blood lipid levels they found that some of the women increased their bone density and actually reversed some of the effects of osteoporosis. This is just one more way to avoid the many problems of menopause. A second study at the University of Illinois (*American Journal of Clinical Nutrition,* v 71, 2000) studied men of widely varying ages with hypercholesterolemia. They gave them soy supplements without any changes in diet or exercise. These men lowered their cholesterol levels significantly in only six weeks.

A Japanese journal (*Daizu Tanakushitsu* v 13, 1992) published a series of articles on soy protein and blood lipids in men and women. These studies were done at Nagoya, Kyushu, Tokai, and Tokushima Universities, and the National Defense Medical College. These studies used different diets and different conditions while giving soy supplements to varying subjects. At all five institutions the conclusions were basically in agreement that modest soy supplementation lowered cholesterol levels and improved the HDL-to-LDL ratios significantly in a short period of time.

At the Dunn Nutrition Center in England (*British Journal of Nutritrion* v 74, 1995) premenopausal women were studied in depth for a full nine months. Of course their cholesterol levels improved when they were fed soy supplements containing isoflavones, but they found other very positive benefits to their health as well. Their hormonal metabolism improved generally, and their menstrual cycles became more regular and less problematic. This was a very unique long term study that shows there are more benefits to soy isoflavones still to be discovered.

The American Heart Nutrition Committee (*Circulation, December 2000*) advised Americans with high cholesterol to add soy protein to their diets. Dr. Erdman at the AHNC said that numerous studies show that soy isoflavones lower TC, LDL, and TG levels, and raise HDL levels. Endorsements from such a prestigious group as this should be heeded.

At Wake Forest University in North Carolina (*Archives of Internal Medicine* v 159, 1999) doctors studied the effects of soy isoflavones on men and women with high cholesterol levels. By giving them a daily supplement over just a two month period they successfully lowered their LDL levels thereby improving their LDL-to-HDL ratios. They also lowered their total cholesterol. This study was extremely professional and very well done.

The Harvard Medical School publishes *The Heart Letter*, which is a very well done monthly report on the studies regarding cures for heart and circulatory problems. In the October 2000 issue they said that studies overwhelmingly prove adding soy to the diet lowers cholesterol, and thereby lowers the risk of heart and artery disease. They went on to say that soy supplements make the blood vessels more elastic, and can actually lower systolic blood pressure (the more important of the two readings). Basic lifestyle changes are usually the only way to lower blood pressure at all, so this is most impressive.

At Wake Forest University again (*Menopause* v 5, 1998) healthy, non-hypercholesterolemic, premenopausal women were given a soy supplement with 34 mg of isoflavones for six weeks, in a classic double blind crossover study. Not only did they lower their total and LDL cholesterol levels but their systolic blood pressure declined as well. They said, "Soy supplementation in the diet of ...women resulted in significant improvements in their lipid and lipoprotein levels, blood pressure and perceived severity of vasomotor symptoms." Remember, these were healthy women who further improved their heart and artery health.

We could go on with study after study on real people given soy isoflavone supplements in clinics around the world, but you see these benefits are established clearly in the medical field. Soy isoflavones improve our blood profiles significantly, improve the quality of our arteries, and are even shown to lower blood pressure. All of these effects can be obtained without any change in diet or exercise. When combined with other proven supplements, a low fat diet and reasonable exercise (such as walking) the effects are even more dramatic.

It has become popular in certain circles, on the Internet, and from some misguided, self-appointed experts to talk about the supposed "dangers" of eating soy foods. This misinformation has become rather popular, despite the fact there are never any valid references to verify their claims of "dangerous side effects" from eating soy foods and taking soy supplements. *All of this propaganda comes from the meat and dairy industries.* It should be obvious that the billions of Asian people, who have eaten soy foods as a basic part of their diets for centuries, never suffer these illusory "side effects". You can see from the many clinical studies that there are never negative side effects from the patients taking these supplements. We have only discussed the benefits of soy isoflavones for blood lipids basically. Entire books have been written about the benefits of soy isoflavones for many other conditions. In fact, new studies are constantly being published, and new benefits are discovered all the time. People are becoming aware that *the real dangers lie in milk and milk products*, and the real benefits are found in soy products. All adults of all races are lactose (milk sugar) intolerant. Milk and dairy consumption is down more every year, especially among African and Asian people, who are the most lactose intolerant. Now grocery stores carry more and more soy milk, soy cheese, soy yogurt, soy cream cheese, soy "meats", various forms of tofu, and other soy products all the time. The dairy interests are understandably upset about so many people switching from dairy products to soy products, and are the ones promoting the disinformation campaign about soy foods. Just realize, this paid propaganda is not from ethical, unbiased scientists.

62

# Chapter 12: Life Style

Aside from the food we eat every day, let's take a quick look at lifestyle. How much exercise do you get every day? Do you drink alcohol? Do you drink coffee? Do you smoke cigarettes? Are you under too much stress? Are you overweight?

*Exercise is the most important life style factor to look at.* Do you do physical work at your job? Do you enjoy any sport like golf or tennis that give you a workout every week? Do you belong to a gym or have workout equipment in your home? Are you a member of an indoor swimming pool? Do you take a walk every day? Walking is the most practical, most effective, and most enjoyable exercise for many people. You can lower your blood lipids as well as lower your blood pressure with no change in diet simply by walking a half hour a day. Studies abound on the cholesterol lowering benefits of any exercise even for young people.

At the University Medical School in Turkey (*Indian Journal of Physiology & Pharmacology* v 43, 1999) it was shown that men of any age who exercised regularly had lower total cholesterol, lower LDL levels, higher HDL levels, less body fat, and all in all less risk for coronary heart disease. At the University of Maryland (*Medical Science Sports Exercise* v 26, 1994) a ten month, long-term study was done on older obese men using a combination of a low-calorie diet and aerobic exercise. Of course the men lost weight and body fat, lowered total, LDL and triglyceride levels, and raised HDL levels. The same university did another long-term, nine month study (*Metabolism & Clinical Experiments* v 48, 1999) on middle-aged, overweight men. This time they put them on the American Heart Association (AHA) diet (which really isn't very strict or hard to follow at all) and had them do aerobic exercise regularly. They got the same results as in the previous study, and the men improved their health very much. At the Center for Adult Diseases in Osaka (*Domyaku Koka* v 21, 1994) doctors took 459 middle aged, healthy men and just had them walk every day. No change in diet, lifestyle or supplements, just walking. They found their HDL levels went up and the risk for coronary heart disease went down almost immediately. At the University of Padua in Italy (*Journal of Sports Medicine* v 31, 1991) healthy young male and female athletes were given either aerobic or resistance exercise. Clear benefits resulted no matter what kind of exercise they did. The usual results of lower TC, LDL, and TG levels, and higher HDL levels were obtained in healthy, young, well-trained athletes. A similar study was done at the University of Vermont (*Metabolism & Clinical Experiment* v. 41, 1992) where the researchers again found whether you do aerobic or resistance exercise it just doesn't matter as you get the same basic cardiovascular benefits. They said," Aerobically trained and resistance trained young males have comparable and favorable cardiovascular disease risk profiles compared with untrained males, and this appears to be related to their low level of adiposity (fat mass) and low intake of dietary fat."

At the University of Pittsburgh (*Journal of Sports Medicine* v 35, 1995) groups of both premenopausal and postmenopausal women were asked to walk every day. The postmenopausal women had an average age of 55 and a whopping 38% body fat! The doctors said, "A single bout of walking has the potential to acutely affect the blood lipid profile of premenopausal as well as postmenopausal women". At Texas A&M University (*Journal of Applied Physiology* v 79, 1995) middle-aged men were given short-term exercise programs with the usual beneficial results. The researchers said, "These data show that a single session of exercise performed by untrained hypercholesterolemic men alters blood lipid and apo-lipoprotein concentrations." Please note, they said just one single session. Exercise is powerful therapy.

You already knew that exercise is good for you and lowers your blood lipids without changing your diet. Think what even daily walking will do when you make some changes in your diet and take proven supplements?

One third of American adults smoke. Smoking is correlated with many major diseases such as various cancers. The biggest and most important heart studies, like the Seven Countries Study, and the Helsinki Study, have repeatedly proven this. Smoking worsens your blood lipid profile, is a major factor for coronary heart disease, is an important factor in many other diseases, and shortens lifespan. The National Cholesterol Education Program published a lengthy report (*Archives of Internal Medicine* v 148,

1988) on all aspects of treating hypercholesterolemia. Examining smoking as a factor, they found that men with the lowest cholesterol levels had only 1.6 deaths per 1,000 if they didn't smoke, but 6.3 deaths if they did. Men with the highest cholesterol levels had 6.4 deaths per 1,000 if they didn't smoke, but a frightening 21.4 deaths if they did. The problem is that nicotine is so addictive it is very hard to stop. There is no reason to quote a list of studies here to show what is already obvious. Smoking is a major factor in heart disease, alters our steroid levels, has countless negative effects on our health, and causes early death. If you want to live a long, healthy life of good quality, and avoid heart and artery disease you have to stop smoking. It is very important to note that when you quit smoking that your health re-covers very quickly, and you soon approach the same level of CHD risk as those who have never smoked. *It is never too late to quit*, and you can quickly reverse most of the damage you've done.

The most impressive study was done on biological twins - one smoked and one didn't (*Thrombosis & Haemotology* v 75, 1996) at the Instituto Scientifico in Italy. The twins who smoked had 13% higher triglycerides, 8% lower HDL levels, as well as an 8% higher white blood cell count (which is a negative) along with other negative changes in their blood parameters. They con-cluded, "Cigarette smoking is associated with an atherogenic lipid profile (i.e. clogs your arteries) and with changes in platelets and white cells potentially reflecting endothelial cell damage." What better proof can you have than identical twins? At the Institute of Biochemistry in Scotland (*European Journal of Clinical Invest-igation* v 23, 1993) the doctors studied healthy men and concluded, "LDL cholesterol, plasma triglycerides, and VLDL (very low density) were found to be substantially increased, and plasma HDL cholesterol decreased in smokers." At the Center for Clinical Studies in Florida (*Contraception* v 44, 1991) doctors studied both pre- and postmenopausal women. It was clear that the women who smoked had lower levels of HDL cholesterol and were at higher risk of CHD – the single biggest killer of women in the U.S. At Osaka Prefectural College in Japan (*Seikatsu Eisei* v 40, 1996) 1,243 Japanese men were studied. They said, "In conclusion, this study of the joint association of cigarette smoking, serum lipid levels, and blood pressure with white blood cell counts as a risk factor for CHD confirming previously reported results..." Please note that the combination of alcohol and nicotine works synergistically together to be much more harmful in effect.

The research showed something fascinating about coffee. One would logically think that it wouldn't matter what kind of coffee you drank, but it very much does. If you drink the regular filtered coffee or instant coffee in moderation (i.e. one or two cups a day) you will suffer less negative effects on your heart. However, if you drink unfiltered, French press, espresso, Turkish and other such types, even two cups a day will affect you very much. This is because the powerful coffee oils cafestol and kaweol are not filtered out. Multiple studies show that the boiled, unfiltered coffee has more harmful effects than the filtered or instant. Some of these studies were done at the Nordic School of Public Health in Sweden, National Institute of Public Health in the Netherlands, and King's College in London. If you are addicted to caffeine, and insist on drinking coffee, always drink the filtered or instant kinds and never more than one cup a day. It's best to give it up.

We come to a much more complex problem with alcohol. Most all countries on earth have a serious problem with alcohol consumption. No other drug on earth causes anywhere near the damage that excessive alcohol consumption does. Every major study has shown that excessive alcohol consumption (i.e. more than two drinks a day or heavy drinking even once a week) is a major risk for coronary heart disease. Ironically, some studies have shown that people who have only one or two drinks a day (and never have more than this) actually have less heart disease better cholesterol levels, and live longer than people who don't drink alcohol at all. *Alcohol, even in moderation, is not part of a healthy lifestyle.* If you only drink one or two drinks a day you may not hurt your blood lipid profile or get more heart disease, but will cause other damage. Drinking more than two drinks a day, or drinking heavily even one day a week will raise your cholesterol, and you'll have a bigger risk of heart and artery disease. You should be aware that even one or two drinks a day has been shown to put your at higher risk for other diseases. Don't listen to the argument that moderate drinking is somehow "good" for your heart and arteries. Alcohol is a poison, not a "French Paradox".

# Chapter 13: Tough Cases

There are a good number of people with genetically high cholesterol and triglycerides, over the 300 level. Such people are at severe risk for all forms of CHD, cancer, diabetes, and premature death. Obviously, they need to do more to lower their blood fats. Here better food choices have to be made, and more supplements and exercise are needed.

There is no cholesterol in any plant. Cholesterol is only found in animals and animal products. People who eat a pure vegetarian diet (no eggs or dairy) consume no cholesterol at all. Such people generally have levels of about 150 mg/dl or less, and every milligram of this is manufactured by their livers from the plant foods they eat. Genetically high people must stop eating all beef, pork, lamb, poultry, eggs, milk, and dairy products. Seafood can be eaten in moderation as a four-ounce daily portion, if you have no allergy. Fatty fish like salmon, swordfish, mackerel, tuna, and catfish (yes, catfish is about 30% fat calories) should be avoided. Low-fat fish such as flounder, grouper, sole, trout, mahi, wahoo, cod, and others are good choices. Shellfish such as crab, scallops, shrimp, and lobster do not raise cholesterol when eaten in moderation. Please read my *Zen Macrobiotics for Americans.*

Vegetable oils contain no cholesterol, but *should be very restricted as well.* Vegetable oils also are generally high in omega-6 fatty acids and low in omega-3 fatty acids. This is another reason to use as little as possible. Americans have an imbalance of omega-6 to omega-3 fatty acids. Flax is the best known source of omega-3 fatty acids, and taking two grams of flax oil is recommended for tough cases. Please refer to Chaper 9: Flax Oil.

Milk and dairy products should be avoided entirely. That includes the low-fat and no-fat varieties, lactose-free, skim milk, and yogurt. Dairy products are full of lactose and casein. There are a variety of very good tasting soy, rice, almond, and oat products to replace them.

It is very important that people with very high blood fats take all four of the "cornerstone supplements"- beta-sitosterol, flax oil, beta glucan and soy isoflavones. It would also be a good idea to double the amount of beta-sitosterol to 600 mg, double the amount of flax oil to 2,000 mg, and double the amount of beta glucan to 400 mg for one year. The guggul gum and soy isoflavones should remain at 250 mg (10% sterones) and 40 mg respectively. Guggul should be discontinued after one year.

Many of the other supplements discussed should also be included in your program. This would include acidophilus, beta carotene, vitamin E, FOS, garlic, L-glutamine, and lecithin. Curcumin, aloe vera, guggul gum, guar gum and citrus pectin for one year only. These supplements are inexpensive, and generally good for your health in many other ways. Take 3 g of TMG (trimethylglycine) daily for one year to rejuvenate and clear out your liver. Good liver function is vital to healthy blood lipid levels.

Hormone balancing in cases like this is no longer an option. As we discuss in Chapters 15 and 16, you must test your basic levels by either using saliva test kits or having your blood diagnosed. DHEA and testosterone are the first ones to measure, but do not take these unless you are proven to be low. Melatonin should be used by people over 40. That can be tested at 3:00 AM with saliva. Transdermal progesterone can be used by both men and women but in different amounts. Pregnenolone should usually be taken by anyone over the age of forty. If estradiol or estrone levels are too high (in men or women), then changes in diet and lifestyle can lower them. Thyroid hormones T3 and T4 should be tested. GH can be used by anyone over the age of 50. This is the only book to talk about the effects of our hormones on our cholesterol and triglyceride levels. Doctors, even endocrinologists, are completely unaware of this, and don't test hormone levels for high blood fats as they should. Cholesterol is the basic hormone from which the sex hormones are made.

Exercise is not an option for tough cases either. You must get more exercise every day than other people. This goes hand in hand with weight loss. People with severely high cholesterol levels need to get down to a normal weight. Fasting one day a week on water is a great help here. Just go from dinner to dinner without eating one chosen day a week without eating. Tough cases need more time, attention and effort to cure.

# Chapter 14: Too Low Cholesterol?

When the "ketogenic" diet was popular, and people ate all the meat and fat they wanted, it was popular to say, "cholesterol doesn't matter". Some even claimed that cholesterol should not be, "too low". This is patently ridiculous of course. A popular life extension magazine states that the optimal range for serum cholesterol is 180 to 200. They further say that cholesterol levels below 180 cause an, "increased risk of mortality". Asinine!

You have seen references to the largest and most comprehensive studies on heart and artery health in the world in this book including the Framingham Study, the 17 Countries Study, and the MRFIT Study. Hundreds of thousands of real people proved that you get benefits all the way down to a level of about 150 mg/dl total serum cholesterol. *TC 150 is the ideal level.*

As we age and reach 60 years we often start losing the ability to synthesize cholesterol. You can find elderly, sickly people who eat a high fat diet, get no exercise, and have very unhealthy lifestyles, yet have rather low cholesterol levels. Therefore, *when we reach old age our cholesterol levels become less accurate in predicting good heart health*. For older people like this you have to look at their cholesterol results in light of how they live. This makes it even more important to eat a low fat diet, exercise, take effective supplements, balance one's hormones, and live a healthy lifestyle generally. Here, we need to distinguish people who have low cholesterol and triglyceride levels due to poor health and poor liver function, compared to those who have low levels due to a low fat diet and healthy lifestyle. Yes, there have been a few studies to show that sickly patients with low cholesterol and unhealthy lifestyles have rare problems like higher specific strokes. *This is due to chronic bad health, poor diet, and the inability to synthesize cholesterol normally. It is certainly not due to low cholesterol per se at all.*

Look at Japan, for example. For centuries the average cholesterol level used to be about 150. This was due to their cultural preference for a low fat diet based on rice, vegetables and seafood. Due to Westernization they now eat much more red

69

meat, poultry, eggs, and even dairy products. These used to be almost unknown there. The average cholesterol level is now about 180, and *heart and artery disease have gone up accordingly*. The Japanese now suffer from far more hypercholesterolemia, high blood pressure, atherosclerosis, aneurisms, strokes, and heart attacks. When 125 million people raise their average cholesterol and suffer a resultant rise in heart and artery disease, the results are clear and inarguable. The rural Japanese do not suffer such problems as they have not adopted the western diet at all. This is especially true of the rural and older Okinawans.

An excellent review from St. Bartholemew's Hospital in London settles this quite well. They went over ten of the largest cohort studies ever done on cholesterol. Every study agreed that *the lower the cholesterol the better,* regardless of any other factors. The authors concluded, "All of them show a similar effect, and none provide any evidence for a threshold below which there ceases to be an effect. The two largest studies provide strong evidence against a threshold over the range of serum cholesterol covered by the studies" (*Atherosclerosis* v 118, 1995).

The high cholesterol crowd loves to refer to an article in the *New England Journal of Medicine* (v 320, 1989). What the doctors really said is that taking all strokes together (hemorrhagic and non-hemorrhagic), the lower your cholesterol level the longer you'll live, *and the less total strokes you'll suffer.* A few sickly, elderly people, with low cholesterol, had slightly more hemorrhagic strokes. However, they were eating high fat, high sugar diets, and their bodies could no longer produce sufficient cholesterol. *Their low levels were due to pathology,* not good diet.

The MRFIT Study of 350,977 men found *the lower your total cholesterol the better*. Men with TC levels of 140 to 159 only had 60 cardiovascular deaths and 15 strokes a year. Men with levels of 220 to 239 had a stunning 562 cardiovascular deaths and 39 strokes. 60 deaths or 562 deaths? The average American has a total cholesterol level over 240, by the way.

People who promote this, "don't let your cholesterol get too low" propaganda are simply trying to justify eating unhealthy high fat foods and lowering the standards of good health.

# Chapter 15: Hormone Balancing

Where else are you going to read about the influence of hormone levels on blood lipid profiles? *Cholesterol is your basic hormone.* Cholesterol is actually the primary hormone from which all our other sex hormones are derived. Did your doctor ever test your basic hormone levels after finding high cholesterol and/or triglycerides? In fact, did your doctor ever suggest testing your basic hormone levels for any reason? Even endocrinologists have no idea that your basic hormones affect blood fat levels. The main thing to understand about our hormones is that *they all work together harmoniously in concert as a team.* Therefore, we need to balance all of the main hormones as much as possible. When one hormone is deficient (or excessive) the others simply cannot function properly. We are going to talk about estrogens, testosterone, T3/T4, DHEA, pregnenolone, insulin (as blood sugar response), progesterone, melatonin, cortisol, as well as growth hormone. *Men and women have exactly the same hormones*, only in different amounts. This could be a very complex and long chapter, but we'll simplify it and not give citations for the hundreds of published studies.

In 2002 the Mississippi Regional Cancer Center published a study, "Hypercholesteremia Treatment: A New Hypothesis" (*Medical Hypotheses* v 59, 2002). This work showed that our general endocrine system has much control over cholesterol and triglycerides. They treated each patient individually with bioidentical DHEA, testosterone, pregnenolone, progesterone, tri-estrogens, and hydrocortisone (cortisol). They normalized blood fats by balancing the hormone levels of their patients with natural hormone replacement therapy. This is unique, professional, and thorough science. It is doctors like this that will lead us into the age of medical enlightenment. A stunning study!

It is a sacred myth in our society that women are somehow "deficient" in estrogen after menopause, and need estrogen supplementation. The truth is that both men and women over 50 in the developed countries are generally excessive in both estradiol and estrone. This is due to many factors such as dietary fat intake, obesity, excessive caloric intake, lack of exercise, and alcohol

71

consumption. One in eight American women will end up with breast cancer, which research shows is a direct effect of high estrogen (estradiol and estrone) levels. One in three will end up with a hysterectomy, which is also a direct effect of excessive estrogen. The current program of routine estrogen supplementation for women is a deadly farce. Women should read my book *No More Horse Estrogen!* Statistics show that ¾ of American men, by age 75, have prostate cancer, and all of them will end up with it if they live long enough. Research reveals that this, too, is a direct effect of excessive estrogen levels. Studies around the world, from institutions such as Columbia University and St. Luke's Hospital, show repeatedly that high estrogen levels in men are associated with cardiovascular disease in general. Men and women should test their free (not bound) levels of estradiol and estrone to see if they are excessive. If you are too high you can *reduce fat intake*, lose weight, exercise, eat more fiber, and stop drinking alcohol. A study at the Pritikin Longevity Center lowered male estrogen levels (along with cholesterol and triglycerides) dramatically in only 26 days(!) simply by giving the men a whole grain, low-fat diet and regular exercise. You can also take proven supplements like 200 mg of di-indolyl methane (DIM) and 1-2 grams of flax oil. Excessive estrogen levels have many other dangerous side effects in both men and women.

Medical doctors, including endocrinologists, don't have the term "estriol" in their vocabulary. Normal pharmacies don't carry it and can't order it. Estriol is the "forgotten estrogen", even though it comprises 80-90% of total estrogen in both men and women. Men are rarely deficient (or excessive) in this. Women should test their estriol levels with a saliva kit. If low use a transdermal cream or gel, or sublingual estriol, but never oral estriol salts.

Both men and women should test their testosterone levels for many reasons. Please read Chapter 7: Cardiovascular Health in my book, *Testosterone Is Your Friend*. Women may be normal, deficient, or excessive in testosterone. Men can only be normal or deficient. Testosterone deficiency is a very important influence in heart and circulatory disease. Men have about ten times more testosterone in their blood than women do. If a woman is excessive she can only lower testosterone levels by diet and lifestyle changes; there are no magic supplements to lower it. Men and women with tested low testosterone levels can use natural prescription testosterone gels or creams, never oral testosterone. Sublingual salts (like enanthate) work well as natural testosterone tastes terrible. Men who are low need about 3 mg daily (4 mg of enanthate sublingually) and women about 150 mcg (200 mcg of enanthate sublingually) in their blood. Never use testosterone unless you have tested yourself and proven you are deficient. The ideal is a youthful level as you had at, say, the age of 30.

DHEA falls generally in both men and women over the age of 40, and is a vital hormone for heart and circulatory health. Women can be excessive, while men are rarely excessive. *Never use DHEA unless you have tested your levels* with either blood or saliva to prove you are low. If you are too high, only diet and life style changes will lower your levels. There are, again, no magic supplements to help you. Men have about twice as much DHEA as women, so women with low levels can try 12.5 mg (half tablets) and men 25 mg daily. DHEA is known as the "life extension hormone" for good reason, and thousands of clinical studies have been done worldwide. At the University of California in San Diego an excellent study concluded DHEA concentration is independently and inversely related to death from any cause and death from cardiovascular disease in men over 50. There are many benefits to keeping a youthful DHEA level throughout life. At Saga Medical School in Japan they found that higher levels of DHEA are related to the favorable lipid and lipoprotein levels in men. What about women? At Medical University Hospital in Germany the doctors found treatment with DHEA raised the initially low serum concentrations of DHEA, testosterone, and androstenedione into the normal range; serum concentrations of SHBG and total cholesterol decreased significantly. At Gifu University in Japan they discovered a favorable effect of DHEA on the lipid profile of Japanese postmenopausal women.

Progesterone is thought of as a female hormone, but it is important for men, too. Progesterone is important for the metabolism of cholesterol. Never use synthetic prescription progestins, as they have many negative side effects and none of the benefits of real progesterone. Use natural USP transdermal progesterone with 800-1000 mg per two ounce jar. Do not use oral progesterone as it is not absorbed well at all. Progesterone is the natural antagonist to excessive estrogen levels, and is very safe and very non-toxic. Both premenopausal women and post-menopausal women may well benefit from using transdermal natural progesterone. Many books have been written on this by such authors as John Lee. Men over fifty can use smaller amounts to protect against estrogen levels, as they usually have higher levels than women of the same age.

You may have never even heard of pregnenolone, but it is the grandmother hormone from which our other sex hormones are derived. *This is the major memory, cognition, and brain hormone.* This is very important to avoid senility, memory loss and Alzheimer's as we age. Take 100 mg of phosphatidyl serine (PS) and 500 mg of acetyl-L-carnitine (ALC) for even better results. Pregnenolone falls quite a bit, after the age of 40, in both men and women, and then stabilizes. Dosages of 25 mg a day for women, and 50 mg a day for men would be reasonable. You can saliva test your levels, or see a doctor for a blood draw. Very little is known about the effects of pregnenolone on our blood lipids, but *it is critical to balance all our hormones together.* Youthful levels are vital to overall hormone balance. Pregnenolone replacement will become much more common as more studies are done, and more is known about it. Common sense logic tells you to keep your pregnenolone at youthful levels throughout life, since it is an intregral part of your endocrine system.

Melatonin is a powerful and miraculous hormone. We are only beginning to understand just how vital it is for our health, well being, and longevity. It is our anti-aging hormone, and decreases from the time we are teenagers until it almost disappears by the time we reach the age of 80. Only recently have studies come to light showing melatonin is vital in the metabolism of cholesterol and triglycerides. This fact is unknown either to the medical profession or the general public.  Studies from the University of Tokyo, University of Seville, Al-Azhar University in Egypt, and Hong Kong Polytechnic University show how vital melatonin is to cholesterol metabolism. They found melatonin  induced a marked protection in terms of decreasing serum cholesterol, LDL, and triglycerides while increasing HDL over 50 percent. Melatonin, secreted by the pineal gland, is the most important anti-aging hormonal factor we know of. You must test this at 3:00 AM by itself with saliva, as melatonin is highest at night when we sleep. If you are over 40 men should take 3 mg and women 1.5 mg (half tabs). *Take this only at night,* and never during the day. This is a very safe and very non-toxic hormone, and a vital part of your supplement program for many, many reasons. Read one of the many books that have been written about it for more information.

Thyroid metabolism is most important for healthy cholesterol levels. You must test your free T3 and free T4, and not your TSH or T3 uptake. Hypothyroidism is epidemic in Westerners over 40. *Look for midrange levels, and do not accept low normal ones.* Synthroid (L-thyroxine) and Cytomel (triiodothyronine) are bioidentical to our own thyroid hormones. If your T3 or T4 level is too high, only diet and life style will lower it. Do not let the doctors butcher or irradiate  your thyroid gland. The best study was from University Hospital in Venezuala where they found 10% of patients with hyperlipidemia were hypothyroid. A review from the University of Nebraska found T4 replacement therapy effectively lowers total cholesterol levels. You can get inexpensive thyroid blood testing on websites like www.healthcheckusa.com without a doctor. Saliva testing will be available in the near future.

Insulin levels per se do not need to be tested, but rather insulin resistance. This is done with a glucose tolerance, or GTT. You drink a cup of glucose solution and wait one hour to get your blood glucose measured, to see how well your insulin responds. Poor response is called "insulin resistance". Blood sugar dys-metabolism, especially diabetes, is closely related to blood lipid conditions. Hyperlididemia is a hallmark of the metabolic syn-drome. *Your fasting blood sugar should be 85 or less.* Your doctor will tell you 100 or less is "fine", but it isn't. Your fasting blood glucose must be *85 or less.* Intake of simple sugars, even honey and maple syrup, is the only cause of excessive fasting blood glucose levels.

Growth hormone is also an important factor in blood fat levels, and growth hormone falls steeply as we age. It is very dif-ficult to get a four sample panel (at 9/1/5/9) over 12 hours. Go by real world results, instead, if you are over 50. Testing IGF-1 levels does *not* work. If you are over the age of 50 you can bet your GH level is low. GH is very overrated because it is expensive. Only real, prescription rhGH (recombinant human growth hormone) works. Research shows all the non-prescription supplements out there claiming to raise growth hormone (no matter how well advertised) are useless. *Life style* keeps your growth hormone level high. Exercise, staying slim, eating less, eating well, fasting regularly, not drinking or smoking, and healthy living generally all work together. Chinese Jintropin® or Hypertropin® are the least expensive. You can use 1 IU daily sublingually, instead of injecting it (but this is not clinically proven). The overwhelming research on using rhGH in the elderly consistently shows improvements in lowering cholesterol and triglycerides levels, as well as raising HDL and lowering LDL. At the world famous NIH in Maryland they concluded that endogenous, nocturnal GH secretion predicts total, LDL, and HDL levels independently. Aarhus University Hospital in Denmark found that GH status is an independent determinant of serum levels of cholesterol and triglycerides in healthy adults. Do not even think of using GH until all your other basic hormones (11 in men and 14 in women) are tested and balanced. *This is the very last hormone to work on.*

We must mention cortisol, the "stress hormone". There is very little information available on supplementing or lowering cortisol and it's relation to blood lipids. The Western Infirmary in Scotland proved that cortisol is integral to cholesterol metabolism in both men and women. High cortisol levels are epidemic in Western societies due to stress, poor diet, and negative life style factors. You can only lower cortisol levels by better food choices, exercise, supplements, general hormone balance, and positive life style changes. A few people are deficient in cortisol, due to adrenal exhaustion, and may benefit from low dose oral hydro-cortisone (the pharmaceutical name for cortisol) therapy. You need to do a four sample comprehensive saliva test (at 9/1/5/9) over twelve hours to see the daily fluctuations.

The next chapter on Home Hormone Testing will tell you how to test most your levels at home with saliva samples accu-rately and inexpensively without a doctor.

# Chapter 16: Home Hormone Testing

---

Medical doctors almost never test their patients for basic hormone levels, regardless of their condition. This includes New Age doctors, holistic practicinoners, naturopaths, and life extension specialists. In the last chapter you saw how critical hormone levels are for your blood lipid levels. Have you ever had a doctor suggest you test your hormone levels for ANY condition? Most all doctors, including endocrinologists, have very little knowledge of hormones, how to test them, or how to supplement low levels. Don't waste your money on testing bound levels of hormones. If you choose a doctor, test your hormone levels, this means multiple blood draws, an expensive office visit, and $100 to $200 per hormone. You still might get back results for bound (unavailable) sex hormones that tell you almost nothing.

Proteins in our bloodstream called SHBG (sex hormone binding globulins) attach themselves to most of our sex hormones making them biologically unavailable. For example, testosterone is usually about 98 percent bound with about 2 percent free (usable) testosterone that actually affects our biological processes. L-thyroxine (T4) is also about 98 percent bound and only about 2 percent biologically available.

For about twenty years now, researchers in clinics have been able to accurately measure hormone levels using saliva samples rather than blood. This was often used in Third World countries, and in the field, due to the lack of available refrigeration for blood samples. The World Health Organization approved this method in the 1990's due to its practicality, accuracy, reliability and low cost. Finally, in the late 1990's, this became available to the general public. You can now buy saliva test kits for estradiol, estrone, estriol, testosterone, androstenedione, DHEA, pregnenolone, cortisol, melatonin, and progesterone among others. You still have to see a doctor to test your insulin, thyroid hormones (T3 and T4) and growth hormone (GH). California and New York have banned this due to pressure from the medical profession. If you live in these states simply use a return address for a friend or relative in another state. There are now Internet sites offering blood testing without a doctor. There are laboratories you can use such as www.healthcheckusa.com to test your blood for free T3, free T4, and TSH for $85 without a doctor at a cooperating clinic.

Saliva testing is a tremendous technological breakthrough in both traditional and holistic medicine, yet very few people and very few doctors are even aware of it. Strangely enough, these are not even sold in pharmacies and drugs stores. The only place to buy saliva hormone test kits is the Internet. Again, this is due to pressure from the medical profession. No matter what your condition, you should know your basic hormone levels. Raise those which are low, and lower those which are excessive. Keeping youthful levels of testosterone, melatonin, progesterone, pregnenolone, T3/T4, DHEA, and growth hormone will add years to your life and life to your years. Even many life extension advocates, that promote the use of these hormones, don't understand that you must test your levels before using them. Almost no one knows what their basic hormone levels are, so they will never enjoy optimal health and lifespan.

For several reasons we no longer list the various laboratories who offer saliva test kits. Just search the Internet for "saliva hormone test kits," and you will find the leading clinics that sell them. Ranges are given for sex and age. Just add high and low range, and divide by 2 to get midrange. Remember, you want the *youthful* levels that you had at about age 30.

These labs generally offer kits that test 1-4 hormones, at about $30-$50 each. Melatonin has to be ordered separately, and tested at 3:00 AM. Vegetarians (and fish eaters) will have lower levels of sex hormones generally. Currently, none of the saliva labs will test T3/T4, insulin, or growth hormone. Time of day is very important for when a sample is taken. Take your samples at the same time every morning (e.g. 8:00 AM) for consistency. Saliva hormone testing is one of the greatest technological advances of the last decade and is now inexpensive, accurate, and practical. Now everyone can test most all their basic hormones at home, inexpensively without a doctor.

# Other Books Available by Safe Goods

| | |
|---|---|
| Testosterone is your Friend – Roger Mason | $ 8.95 |
| The Natural Prostate Cure – Roger Mason | $ 7.95 |
| Zen Macrobiotics for Americans – Roger Mason | $ 7.95 |
| The Minerals You Need – Roger Mason | $ 4.95 |
| What is Beta Glucan – Roger Mason | $ 4.95 |
| No More Horse Estrogen – Roger Mason | $ 7.95 |
| The Natural Diabetes Cure – Roger Mason | $ 7.95 |
| Lower Blood Pressure Without Drugs-Roger Mason | $ 8.95 |
| Cancer Disarmed Expanded | $ 7.95 |
| Atlantis Today- The USA | $ 9.95 |
| Live Disease Free | $ 9.95 |
| Rx for Computer Eyes | $ 8.95 |
| Eye Care Naturally | $ 8.95 |
| 2010 Airborne Prophecy | $ 16.95 |
| Overcoming Senior Moments | $ 9.95 |
| The Secrets of Staying Young | $ 9.95 |
| ADD, The Natural Approach | $ 4.95 |
| The ADD and ADHD Diet | $ 9.95 |

*For a complete listing of books visit our web site:*
*www.safegoodspub.com to order or call (888) 628-8731*
*For a free catalog (888) NATURE-1*

## Seven Steps to Natural Health

With these seven steps you can cure "incurable" illnesses like cancer, diabetes, heart disease, and others naturally without drugs, surgery, or chemotherapy. These are seven vital steps to take if you want optimum health and long life. Do your best to do all of them. The only step to add would be prayer or meditation.

- An American macrobiotic whole grain based diet is central to everything. Diet cures disease; everything else is secondary.

- Proven supplements are powerful when you're eating right. There are only about twenty scientifically proven supplements for those over forty, and eight for those under forty.

- Natural hormone balance is the third step. There are fourteen basic hormones. You can do this inexpensively without a doctor.

- Exercise is vital, even if it is just a half hour of walking a day. Whether it is aerobic or resistance you need to exercise regularly.

- Fasting is the most powerful healing method known to man. Just fast from dinner to dinner on water one day a week. Join our monthly Young Again two day fast. The fasting calendar is at www.youngagain.org on the last weekend of every month.

- No prescription drugs, except *temporary* antibiotics or pain medication during an emergency. (There are rare exceptions such as insulin for type 1 diabetics who have no operant pancreas.)

- The last step is to limit or end any bad habits such as alcohol, coffee, recreational drugs, or desserts. You don't have to be a saint, but you do have to be sincere.